MW00745327

APR 7 2000

REFERENCE LIBRARY

Springer Series on **Behavior Therapy and Behavioral Medicine**

Series Editor: Cyril M. Franks, Ph.D.
Advisory Board: John Paul Brady, M.D., Robert P. Liberman, M.D.,
Neal E. Miller, Ph.D., and Stanley Rachman, Ph.D.

Series volumes no longer in print are listed on the following page.

Out of Print Titles

The Psychological Management OF Chronic Pain

A Treatment Manual

Second Edition

WORKPLACE SAFETY
& INSURANCE BOARD
RECEIVED

APR 7 2000

REFERENCE LIBRARY

H. Clare Philips, PhD

Stanley Rachman, PhD

*Springer Series on Behavior Therapy
and Behavioral Medicine*

First edition published, 1988

Copyright © 1996 by Springer Publishing Company, Inc.

All rights reserved

No part of this publication may be reproduced, stored in a retrieval system, or transmitted in any form or by any means, electronic, mechanical, photocopying, recording, or otherwise, without the prior permission of Springer Publishing Company, Inc.

Springer Publishing Company, Inc.
536 Broadway
New York, NY 10012-3955

Cover design by Tom Yabut
Production Editor: Pam Ritzer

98 99 00 / 5 4 3   Third Printing

Library of Congress Cataloging-in-Publication Data

Philips, Clare.
    The psychological management of chronic pain : a treatment manual / H. Clare Philips, Stanley Rachman. — 2nd ed.
      p. cm. — (Springer series on behavior therapy and behavioral medicine)
    Includes bibliographical references and index.
    ISBN 0-8261-6111-1
    1. Chronic pain—Psychological aspects. 2. Behavior therapy.
I. Rachman, Stanley. II. Title. III. Series: Springer series on behavior therapy and behavioral medicine (Unnumbered) [DNLM:
    1. Pain— therapy. 2. Chronic Disease. 3. Pain—psychology.
    4. Behavior Therapy.   WL 704 P554p 1996]
RB127.P49   1996
616.0472—dc20
DNLM/DLC
for Library of Congress   95–39060
                                        CIP

Printed in the United States of America

Acknowledgments

The people who contributed most to the evolution of this training method are the many chronic pain patients with whom we have worked during the last few years. Their comments, criticisms, and courage have been inspiring and helpful.

We are indebted to many people for their advice and assistance, but foremost among these are Ronald Melzack and Patrick Wall, whose contribution to understanding the psychology of pain is unsurpassed, and whose ideas provided the inspiration for this book. The advice of Caroline Carson (physical therapist), Linda Hensman and Lynn Pollock (pharmacists), and Dr. Ian Tsang (consultant physician) have been invaluable. Holly Jeffares and Adam Radomsky provided valuable assistance in preparing the manuscript.

Clare Philips, PhD, is a clinician-researcher specializing in the psychology of pain. Her research into the nature and treatment of chronic headaches broke new ground, and she made important contributions to the early development of programs for the psychological management of chronic pain. She is the author of two books and numerous articles.

Stanley J. Rachman, PhD, is a professor in the Psychology Department of the University of British Columbia, and a Fellow of the Royal Society of Canada. He has conducted clinical research on many aspects of emotion, including the emotional component in chronic pain, memory for pain, and the overprediction of pain. He is the author of eight books and numerous articles.

Contents

PART II: Treatment

Preface

The reception of the First Edition of this book was encouraging, and we were particularly gratified by reports from patients who were helped by participating in the pain-management program. The need for a revised and expanded Second Edition arises from the accumulation of new knowledge about pain, the enlightening infusion of cognitive psychology into clinical psychology, and of course the need to bring the material and methods up to date.

The book provides the clinician with a practical guide to the management of chronic pain problems. It describes a program that comprises psychological and associated methods of inducing cognitive-behavioral changes, and is based on a persuasive neurophysiological model of pain: the Gate Control Model. An important feature of the program is its practicality for the busy clinician, faced by an ever-increasing number of referrals for alleviating chronic pain. The manual has been prepared for cognitive-behaviorally trained clinical psychologists wishing to undertake the management of this major medical psychological problem. Many clinicians were trained prior to the development of specific techniques for the management of chronic pain, but their general skills are readily applicable to pain problems.

This manual provides the structure and the detailed information to enable them to move with confidence into this expanding area of psychological modification. The pain management program was developed to meet the needs of a psychology department within a general hospital that was receiving large numbers of referrals for chronic pain management. The hospital setting provided an excellent milieu for the progressive expansion of the program to include the consultative support of a physician, pharmacist, and physiotherapist. Referrals came from a broad range of physicians (rheumatologists, orthopedic surgeons, oral surgeons, general practitioners, urologists). Their patients reported chronic pain problems that had endured for an average of eight years prior to their referral to the psychology department. Patients had visited medical specialists over the years, without finding satisfactory solutions to their difficulties. The effectiveness of the program encouraged the publication of this method. The results, which have been found to endure for up to a year posttreatment, suggest that a psychologically directed approach can be lastingly effective.

The organization of this book into sessional components allows the clinician flexibility in the application of this method. The method can be adapted to the needs of particular patients, or the demands of groups, while maintaining a coherent structure in which to work. Just as the patient is encouraged to experiment with strategies, clinicians are encouraged to explore the efficacy of various techniques which they teach to patients.

The structured approach can be established comparatively easily, and operates in a cost-efficient manner. The recommended group format allows six to eight cases to be treated effectively by one professional, in approximately 14 hours of therapeutic time. Despite the group framework in which it has been evolved, the program can be used equally well for the treatment of individual cases.

In order to keep the manual in a usable form, supportive material has been kept to a minimum and suggested readings provided at the conclusion of each chapter. In addition, separate workbooks are available from the publisher for the patients to use. Those interested in the experimental and/or clinical background of the method, or who become inspired to explore the strategies and techniques further, are advised to follow up on the suggested readings, many of which are excellent. This text provides the background for pain management, a detailed explanation of methods and of strategies, as well as the approach to selection and to treatment evaluation. In addition, it provides some answers to problems that may arise. Other professionals working with chronic pain patients will also find this a useful resource (physical therapists, occupational therapists, social workers, general practitioners, neurologists, rehabilitation specialists, nurses, etc.).

In this new edition we have placed increasing emphasis on the cognitive components of treatment, and expanded the introductory section to include a fuller description of the ''new'' psychology of pain, memory for pain, the overprediction of pain, pain-related cognitions, and how they are measured. The practical orientation of the first edition has been retained. It is our hope and expectation that health-care professionals who provide treatment, care, and comfort for pain sufferers will find the program usable and effective.

The component organization of the program also provides a usable structure for research. It is hoped that the details provided in this manual will lead to replication, assessment, and development of the techniques described. The overall efficacy of this approach calls for such steps to be undertaken, and this manual will provide the source material for research studies in independent settings by trained clinicians. The next few decades will be important for those involved in pain management. Recognition of the potency of psychological factors in the management of chronic pain is now undisputed. Attention can justifiably be turned to the intriguing issues of matching techniques with persons, of demonstrating the potency of techniques in relation to the intensity and type of pain, of developing techniques to prevent the insidious growth of chronic pain problems, and of evaluating the short- and long-term effects of pain management strategies.

Patient's Manual

In order to integrate and synchronize the treatment tactics used in the therapy sessions with the practice that the patient carries out between sessions, we recommend that each patient use his or her own workbook— the *Patient's Manual*. In the Manual a separate chapter is provided for each treatment session, thereby encouraging the patient to integrate the treatment and practice sessions in a simple, easily used format. The chapters contain all of the key information provided in each session, plus advice and reminders, and simple recording charts. In this way the tasks of the therapist and the patients can be closely synchronized. The *Patient Manual* also enables patients to keep a detailed record of their personal progress. The manuals are available from the publisher of this Treatment Manual, Springer Publishing Company, 536 Broadway, New York, New York, 10012.

PART I

The Self-Management Approach

Introduction

The first part of this book concentrates on the theoretical and practical issues that underlie the self-management approach to chronic pain. Recognition of the importance of psychological factors in modulating pain levels has allowed clinicians to develop psychological methods for improving the self-management of pain problems. The structure, nature, and key parameters of the approach are detailed, and issues relating to assessment and selection of patients are clarified.

CHAPTER 1

Introduction

THE EFFECTS OF CHRONIC PAIN

Chronic pain is a major health problem in our society. In the United States, the financial cost of chronic pain is estimated to be as high as $90 billion per year. This figure was calculated by adding the cost of compensation claims, time off work, medication, disability allowances, etc., all of which arose from chronic pain problems. This enormous sum, no doubt larger now and still growing, emphasizes the magnitude of the problem, but does not include the distressing, erosive and sometimes catastrophic effects of continuing pain upon the sufferer's life. Even when the distress and pain are focused (e.g., in the lower back or in the jaw), the effects are seldom circumscribed. A growing helplessness, depression, or fear may dominate people as they face the implications of their disabilities and their reduced capacities to earn a living or raise children. A growing sense of frustration and anger is understandable in any person who has come to believe that medicine will have answers for any pain problem. Frequently, there is a marked development of avoidance of activity, exercise, intimacy, and pleasurable activities. The person becomes increasingly isolated, with disruption of relationships and growing physical disability. Pain often provokes emotions and moods that can exacerbate pain. The fear of a worsening of the pain problem often leads to withdrawal and the consequent development of disuse syndrome and muscular weakness. Multiple surgeries (e.g., to the back), in an attempt to rectify the person's suffering, may lead to increasing muscle scarring and complex iatrogenic problems. Attempts to bring even temporary relief to the sufferer through drugs may lead to dependency and debilitating side-effects.

In summary, the person suffering from a continuing pain problem may well react in a manner that exacerbates the difficulties as vicious circles are established. The effects of a chronic pain problem may expand with the years, establishing behavior that leaves the person increasingly impotent and unable to control the escalating problems. The bleak effects of continuing pain can occur regardless of the type of pain they experience. The psychological correlates of pain are similar, whether it be lower back pain, facial pain, headache, leg pain, pelvic floor pain, and so forth. Because of the important similarities between types of chronic pain, psychological management can be effective, regardless of the specific locus of the pain. In due course, we hope to see the development of increasingly specialized techniques for concentrating on particular aspects of each type of pain, but at present our understanding of pain management has not reached this level of sophistication. At this stage it is already evident that once a pain problem becomes chronic, psychological factors are of increasing importance in the understanding and management of the problem.

PSYCHOLOGICAL INFLUENCES ON CHRONIC PAIN

There often is a lag between the introduction of a new theoretical framework and the elaboration of its practical consequences. This type of lag is demonstrated in an exemplary manner by the current thinking and practice on the subject of chronic pain. Some years ago, it became evident that there were a number of experimental and clinical findings that could not be explained by the established medical model of pain. The traditional view was based upon the view that the amount of pain a person felt was roughly proportional to the extent and site of the putative tissue damage. Although a useful framework for dealing with acute injury, it was ill-adapted for explaining pain that continues after tissue healing. The weaknesses of the traditional approach to pain are described in Chapter 2.

The Gate Control Model

In recognition of the weaknesses of the traditional approach, Melzack and Wall (1965) introduced a fresh model, the Gate Control, that has proved to be extremely helpful in explaining clinical and experimental phenomena, but unfortunately the theory's influence on medical practitioners and the general public has been limited. (See Melzack, 1993; Melzack & Wall, 1988; Wall & Melzack, 1989.)

The Gate Control Model acknowledges that chronic pain is a complex phenomenon entailing not only aversive sensory and affective experiences, but also cognitive-behavioral changes and adjustments in motivation, in mood, and in cognitions. The importance of psychological factors in mediating pain experience, in exacerbating or ameliorating pain problems, and in influencing pain behavior is fully acknowledged by the new model, but not yet elaborated. Pain perception is influenced not only by messages moving up to the brain to be interpreted, but it also is modulated by descending messages from the brain that can attenuate or even block ascending messages under certain circumstances. Physiological mechanisms were postulated that are influenced by descending messages from the brain, and, in turn, affect the influence of ascending messages. This model draws attention to the importance of considering and exploiting central, or descending, influences on pain perception and tolerance. In doing so, it helps explain the remarkable effect that psychological factors can have in modulating pain, as well as the vicious circles that can develop for chronic pain sufferers who become distressed and/or depressed by prolonged pain. This explanation is readily understandable to the chronic pain patient, and gives a legitimacy to their suffering. In addition, it acts as a motivation to mobilize psychological factors in order to limit and to reduce their pain problem.

THE SELF-MANAGEMENT APPROACH

The ideas utilized in developing this program of chronic pain management were derived from a number of sources, but most importantly, the approach was directly inspired by the invaluable writings of Melzack and Wall

(1965, 1988). The recommendations from these and many other psychologists writing on the subject of chronic pain were integrated into a framework that was derived from the Melzack-Wall Gate Control Model. In addition to these academic influences, the program has been substantially shaped by the experience of dealing with countless chronic pain patients over a number of years. Their reactions to treatment and their attempts to evolve tactics that would modulate their pain proved invaluable in developing techniques that could be taught to other patients. Finally, this program has been strongly influenced by the authors' training and experience in clinical psychology from a cognitive-behavioral perspective. Many methods utilized in clinical psychology for treating other problems are applicable to the management of chronic pain and have provided useful tools for dealing with specific issues that arise in the management of associated problems (e.g., excessive anxiety, depressive reactions, etc.).

The approach that has evolved has many characteristics in common with self-management programs that have been developed throughout North America during the last decade. It is innovative to the extent that, over a short series of training sessions, persons are encouraged to gain control over their pain problems, using a psychologically directed perspective.

The crucial emphasis of this method is the importance it places on the patient's participation in learning management techniques that will help him or her control and, therefore, minimize pain. Such an approach can be distinguished from any attempt to ''cure'' the patient. The term *cure* comes directly from the medical model and is considered inappropriate. Patients are persuaded to become the active directors of their own improvement, rather than passive recipients of medical treatments. The ways in which they are taught to manage pain are derived from the Gate Control Model, exploiting the inhibitory influences that cognitive, emotional, and behavioral factors can have upon pain experience. Consistent with this, patients become minor experts on the effect of chronic pain upon various aspects of their life and on the power they can exert in modulating its influence. A sense of control develops, and remarkable shifts in attitude often occur.

Three examples illustrate the types of changes that patients can make in their pain problem as a consequence of attending treatment sessions. They have been chosen to illustrate the extent of the adjustment and the manner in which these adjustments increment over time, as patients improve their ability to utilize the strategies.

Case 1

A 47-year-old woman reported constant low back pain problem from which she had been suffering for 10 years. Periodically, she was totally incapacitated by episodes of stronger, sharper pain, and at these times was unable to do housework or continue her job.

She improved gradually during treatment, becoming increasingly confident in her capacity to manage pain episodes. At one-year follow-up, she reported that she was no longer experiencing significant pain and rated herself as having complete control over it. Using most of the strategies taught to her, she could undertake all activities except vacuuming. She reported herself as no longer feeling that she had a pain problem, had ceased taking analgesics, had not taken time off work since the completion of treatment, and was seeking no further help with pain.

Case 2

A 37-year-old married woman was referred because of multiple chronic pains that led her to give up work and retire to a life of almost constant resting. She had been incapacitated by the pain for five years. During treatment, she made steady progress, which was maintained after completion of the program. At one-year follow-up, she arrived dressed for professional work. During the follow-up period, she had undertaken and completed a real estate training course and was working full-time. She described herself as having ''very little problem to speak of.'' She used the strategies she had learned as a part of her manner of living and felt no need for further treatment. She spontaneously reported large increases in self-esteem, both at work and at home, and an improvement in her relationship with her family.

Case 3

A 32-year-old student and part-time teacher was referred for severe and often incapacitating headaches. She was using large doses of Fiorinal®

C1/2 (up to an average of 6–7 per day) with additional Tylenol®, codeine, Gravol®, and aspirin.

At one-year follow-up, she was using no medication to control her headaches, and their impact on her life had dropped dramatically. The continuous pattern that she had experienced was broken, and she was experiencing only occasional migraines, usually related to her menstrual cycle and particularly when personal pressures were high. When headaches did occur, they were less intense. She estimated her control over pain to have increased by at least 40%, and was not seeking further help with her headaches.

It is hoped that a program such as the one described in this manual will go some way toward bridging the gap that has developed between theory and practice. As this gap is crossed, doctors and patients will begin to demand psychological help in the management of pain problems that persist after tissue has healed.

SUGGESTED READINGS

Blanchard, E. B., & Andrasik, F. (1985). *The management of chronic headache: A psychological approach.* New York: Pergamon Press.

Bonica, J. J. (Ed.). (1990). *The management of pain.* Malvern, PA: Lea & Febiger.

Fordyce, W. E. (1976). *Behavioral methods for chronic pain and illness.* St. Louis: Mosby.

Melzack, R., & Wall, P. (1988). *The challenge of pain.* Harmondsworth, UK: Penguin Books.

Turk, D. C., Meichenbaum, D., & Genest, M. (1983). *Pain and behavioral medicine: A cognitive behavioral perspective.* New York: Guilford Press.

Wall, P., & Melzack, R. (Eds.). (1989). *Textbook of pain (2nd ed).* Livingston, Edinburgh.

Weisenberg, M. (1980). Understanding pain phenomena. In S. Rachman (Ed.), *Contributions to medical psychology* (Vol. 2, pp. 70–111). Elmsford, NY: Pergamon Press.

Weisenberg, M. (1987). Psychological intervention for the control of pain. *Behavior Research & Therapy, 25,* 301–312.

CHAPTER 2

The Nature of Pain

Before describing the details of the Program, recent developments in the psychology of pain are reviewed.

The experience of pain is a complex psychological phenomenon in which the meaning of the pain has a powerful influence on the duration and intensity of the associated distress. A familiar pain that is interpreted as harmless is more easily tolerated and less distressing than an unfamiliar pain that is interpreted as a sign of a potentially serious illness or injury. A person who interprets the pain in his/her chest as familiar indigestion brought on by spicy foods is well able to tolerate the discomfort. A comparable pain in the chest experienced for the first time by someone with a fear of sudden death may be interpreted as extremely dangerous, and hence become intensely distressing and intolerable. "The amount and quality of pain we feel are also determined by our previous experiences and how well we remember them, by our ability to understand the cause of the pain and to grasp its consequence" (Melzack & Wall, 1988, p. 15). The experience of pain, and what we do about it, is essentially a psychological phenomenon, and not merely an automatic reaction to injury or illness. Central influences flow down from the brain to block, amplify, delay, or complicate our reactions to injuries and illnesses (Melzack, 1993).

It must be remembered however, that in many circumstances, especially those involving acute and localized injuries, the pain is indeed a direct reflection of the injury and proportional to the severity of the injury, just as described in the traditional theory of pain. In other circumstances, particularly those in which the pain is chronic and variable, the relationship between the injury/illness (if any) and the pain is complex and often puzzling.

For a considerable period it was believed that the relationship between pain and injury is direct and simple. The fundamental idea, embodied in the classical "specificity theory," was that pain is a direct result of injury. Furthermore, it was believed that the pain reflects the injury; the intensity of the pain reflects the seriousness of the injury, the duration of the pain is determined by the nature of injury and the time taken for healing to occur, and the site of the pain corresponds to the site of injury. It followed from these beliefs that any pain experienced in the absence of a detectable injury must be imaginary or suspect, and that there should be a close match between the seriousness of the injury and the amount of pain experienced. Once the healing process was completed the pain should disappear.

The experience of pain was construed as an exchange. Injuries set off impulses that arc transmitted directly up the spinal cord to the brain where they are interpreted. Impulses then flow back down to the site of the injury and a direct response, such as withdrawal, is triggered.

In many cases of injury, especially those of an acute and severe kind, the ideas incorporated in the specificity theory are still applicable, but it has become evident that the idea of a simple and direct relationship between pain and injury, is mistaken. There are numerous and important exceptions to this view, and recognition of these exceptions and their significance, finally led to the introduction of a fresh theory of pain, Melzack and Wall's "gate control theory," described in Chapter 1. Important exceptions to the main assumptions of the specificity theory are set out in Table 2.1.

To begin, there are many important and common instances of genuine pain being experienced in the absence of any identifiable injury. For example, in the majority of cases of low back pain, in which the person experiences intense and recurrent pain which can be incapacitating, thorough clinical investigations fail to reveal any detectable cause of the pain; that is, no injury is detectable (Melzack & Wall, 1988).

TABLE 2.1   Pain With and Without Injury

---

1.   **PAIN WITHOUT IDENTIFIABLE INJURY**
      e.g., cases of low back pain, pelvic pain, tension headache, persisting phantom limb pain

2.   **INJURY WITHOUT PAIN**
      e.g., sporting injuries, combat casualties, self-injurious acts, masochism, unusual states, hypnosis, fire-walkers

2(a). **INJURY/DYSFUNCTION WITHOUT PAIN**
      e.g., spinal abnormalities, such as protrusions, without pain

3.   **INJURY AND PAIN DISPROPORTIONATE**
      e.g., cases of chronic facial pain, low back pain, ritual injuries inflicted by dervishes and other sects, minimal pain despite severe wounds in combat troops

4.   **DISJUNCTIONS IN TEMPORAL RELATION BETWEEN PAIN AND INJURY**
      e.g., cases of chronic post-operative pain, dental pains, phantom limb pain, delayed onset of pain after traumatic injuries

5.   **TREATMENT CONUNDRUMS**
      e.g., surgical failures, brief analgesia producing lasting pain relief, hypnosis, placebos

6.   **QUALITIES OF PAIN TOO COMPLEX FOR SPECIFICITY THEORY**
      e.g., memory too complex, pain comprises of at least three dimensions (affective, sensory, evaluative)

Pelvic pain, another common and unpleasant disorder, also defies the search for identifiable injuries; commonly, there are none, but the pain is not to be denied. The most common form of headache, so-called "tension headache," occurs recurrently and can become extremely intense, but there is no underlying injury and scant evidence of abnormalities or dysfunctions (Philips, 1983). These headaches may be the result of unadaptive muscular or vascular activities, but the precise cause remains unknown.

Perhaps the most remarkable and puzzling form of pain occurring in the absence of injury is the phenomenon of phantom limb pain (Melzack, 1989). In these cases, the person continues to experience sensations, and even pain, in a limb that has been removed during surgery or lost in the course of an accident. Typically, the person continues to feel the presence of the limb and frequently these sensations are accompanied by unremitting burning pain. Phantom limb pains can persist for prolonged periods, even years, and well after the injury has healed. Furthermore, persistence of this pain in the absence of continuing injury, cannot be attributed to irritation of the remaining nerve supply because surgical treatments in which the nerve supply to the affected area is deliberately severed, seldom eliminates the phantom limb pain.

In addition to these common examples of pain occurring in the absence of detectable injury, there are many examples in which injuries fail to produce pain. One of the most commonly encountered of these examples of injury without pain are found in sporting activities. It is commonly the case that an injury, even a serious injury, which is incurred during the course of an exciting or distracting game will produce no pain, at least during the conduct of the game itself. In many instances pain begins to appear some hours or days after the game has been completed, but in other examples the injury, even a break, is not accompanied by pain.

But the most remarkable examples of injuries occurring without accompanying pain are seen in combat casualties. The first person to fully acknowledge the important significance of these combat casualties was a physician in the U.S. medical corps, Dr. H. K. Beecher (1959). He described cases of soldiers who incurred wounds, even very severe wounds, during World War II battles but reported that they had little or no pain and displayed little of the behavior that is characteristic of painful experiences. Similar observations have been made in other countries. A remarkable number of these wounded soldiers felt no need for powerful pain-killing medications, in contrast to patients whom Dr. Beecher had seen in his pre-war civilian practice, who reported and exhibited intense pain even after comparatively minor injuries and invariably requested pain-reducing medications.

Other examples of injuries occurring without accompanying pain include uncommon but distressing examples of self-mutilation. A small number of people who suffer from serious psychological disorders and who endure extraordinarily intense periods of psychological tension find that they can obtain temporary relief from their distress by injuring themselves. For example, one of our patients discovered almost incidentally that she could gain some relief from unendurable tension by cutting herself in the arm, or later, in the leg or stomach. She was an intelligent and creative woman whose psychological problems were deep and long-lasting, and as the episodes of tension and subsequent cutting increased in frequency, the scarring on her arms and legs became so extensive that it was difficult for medical staff to stitch the wounds. As in other similar cases, the patient made it clear that the cuts which she inflicted upon herself, often quite deep, produced no pain, but rather a sense of relief. This was not because she was incapable of experiencing pain, but rather that in these abnormal psychological states of tension, the injuries produced no pain. Interestingly, when she had to have the stitches removed days or weeks after the cut had been treated, she usually experienced pain. During the episodes of severe tension she had no pain, but when the tension passed, she again felt appropriate pain.

Another set of examples of injury occurring without pain, but accompanied rather by a sense of pleasure, is seen in cases of masochism. In these instances, the person solicits punishment, even of a severe kind, up to and including flogging or beating, and experiences pleasure, usually sexual pleasure, and no trace of pain. Additionally, injuries that are incurred during unusual states, such as religious trances, are accompanied by a state of ecstasy rather than pain. Some years ago we observed a fire-walking ceremony that was part of a ritual conducted by a religious Hindu sect. Prior to walking across the burning coals there was a long preparatory period during which the participants worked themselves into a state of religious frenzy. At the critical moment, while they were in this unusual and elevated psychological state, they ran across the bed of burning coals and experienced religious fulfillment and no pain.

Lastly, there is the commonly demonstrated phenomenon of pain that is blocked or completely inhibited during hypnosis even when the subject is prodded with a sharp instrument or exposed to an extremely hot stimulus, such as fire. Despite the evidence of injury, the hypnotic subject will experience no pain, either during the trance or after.

Examples of injury or abnormality *without pain* were encountered in the continuing attempts to understand the elusive nature of low back pain, and are important not only because of their theoretical significance but also because of the extensity of the problem. Jensen, Turner, and Romano (1994, p. 69) estimated the lifetime prevalence of low back pain at approximately 80%, with 31 million Americans experiencing low back pain at any given time. They go on to say that "in the United States, low back pain is second only to the common cold as the reason patients cite for seeking medical care" (p. 69). The examples are also of clinical importance in illustrating that a simple equation between low back pain and some abnormality or injury is untenable. Jensen and colleagues carried out MRI (Magnetic Resonance Imaging) on 92 asymptomatic people (i.e., without low back pain). The scans were read independently by two neuroradiologists who were unaware of the status of the subjects. In addition, abnormal scans from 27 people with back pain were mixed in randomly with the scans from the asymptomatic people. No less than 38% of the asymptomatic subjects had "an abnormality of more than one intervertebral disk" (p. 69); and Jensen et al. concluded that "given the high prevalence of these findings and of back pain, the discovery by MRI of bulges or protrusions in people with low back pain may frequently be coincidental" (p. 69). Moreover, 67% of the 27 people who were 50 years or older had multiple abnormalities, compared to the smaller number of 27% for the younger subjects. The significance of these findings is emphasized by the remarkable fact that "only 36% of those examined had a normal disk at all levels" (p. 72). Given a base rate of this size casts a new and radically different light on the routine use of scans for reaching diagnostic and therapeutic decisions.

Similar results were reported by Boden and colleagues (1990) who carried out MRI scans of 67 people who had never experienced low back pain or associated problems. The scans were interpreted independently by three specialists who were unaware of the presence or absence of clinical symptoms in the subjects. They found that one third of the subjects had "a substantial abnormality" (Boden, Davis, Dina, Patronas, & Wiesel, 1990, p. 403), and among the people who were 60 years or older, the findings were abnormal in approximately 57% of the scans. There was degeneration or bulging of a disk in at least one lumbar level in all but one of the subjects above the age of 60, and among 35% of the subjects between 20 and 39 years of age. They concluded that abnormalities on MRI scans "must be strictly correlated with age and any clinical signs and symptoms before operative treatment is contemplated'' (p. 403). Boden et al. (1990) found that 30% of their asymptomatic subjects had a "major abnormality on a MRI of the lumbar spine" (p. 406). This is another piece of evidence to be taken into account when calculating base rates of abnormality in low back pain. Jensen, Brant-Zawadzki et al. (1994) reported comparable findings.

The detection of significant spinal abnormalities in asymptomatic patients is not confined to results from Magnetic Resonance Imaging. In a sample of asymptomatic people over the age of 40, Wiesel et al. (1984) found an average of 50% of abnormal findings on the basis of CAT scans (Computer-Assisted Tomography). Among the entire sample of 57 scans, 35% of those taken from asymptomatic patients were interpreted as being abnormal. The results from this CAT study must be regarded with caution, however, because of the considerable disagreement between the three neuroradiologists who interpreted the scans independently and blindly. Surprisingly, they were in total agreement in only 6 of the 52 CAT scans of asymptomatic patients rated by all three raters (but the three were in full agreement on the six scans from patients who had significant back pain). The wider significance of these disagreements in interpreting the CAT scans should be noted, but will not be elaborated on at present.

Contrary to the idea that there is a close correspondence between the seriousness and the extent of the injury and the amount of pain experienced, there are numerous exceptions in which a minor injury is followed by very severe pain, or major injuries in which the accompanying pain is trivial. There are numerous cases of chronic facial pain in which the initiating event is a comparatively minor injury but the pain, which can be intense, persists for months or even years. Causalgia is intense, burning pain in the area that is served by a damaged nerve, but persists well after the healing process has been completed (Melzack & Wall, 1988). Unfortunately, direct treatment of the injured nerve supply, or even the surgical interruption of the nerve supply, is not a reliable way of dealing with the problem. Certainly, the severity and duration of causalgia is entirely disproportionate to the original injury.

Contrary to the fundamental belief that there should be, or always is, a close relationship between the time which the injury occurs and the emergence of the pain, there is abundant evidence of exceptions to this relationship. There are numerous cases of chronic postoperative pain, which continues for months or years after the surgical injury has healed. Chronic dental pains provide another set of examples, as does phantom limb pain referred to earlier. In an interesting study conducted at the Emergency Rooms in the Montreal General Hospital, Melzack and Wall (1982) observed the relationship between the occurrence of an injury and the onset of pain. Of the 138 patients who were alert and rational, 37% stated that they did not feel pain at the time of incurring the acute injury. The majority reported that pain had begun within an hour of the injury but the delays were as long as 9 hours or more in some patients. Of the 46 patients whose injuries were limited to the skin (cuts, burns, abrasions), no less than 53% had a pain-free period. Even when there is a correspondence between injury and pain, the effects are not always immediate.

There are several treatment effects that are difficult to understand in terms of the specificity theory with its assumption of a direct and simple connection between injury and illness. In numerous cases of chronic pain, surgical interventions are surprisingly disappointing; even if the supposed transmission between the site of injury and the central nervous system is surgically interrupted, the pain may nevertheless persist. The experience of pain is determined to a considerable extent by events in the upper centers of the central nervous system, and these influences are complex. So for example, it is common for people to achieve relief from pain by taking inert, nonactive medications (placebos). These so-called "nonspecific" effects are pervasive and can be powerful (Turner, Deyo, Loeser, von Korff, & Fordyce, 1994). Nonspecific therapeutic effects can even be obtained after "erroneous" surgery. A strong expectation that taking the tablet will provide relief is sufficient to bring about psychological changes that result in a reduction or elimination of the pain. The potential power of higher level nervous system functioning is also seen in the capacity of hypnosis to block pain. These reductions in pain can occur irrespective of the presence or absence of any injury.

Finally, it has become abundantly clear that the psychological qualities of pain are far too complex to be understood in terms of a simple and direct connection between injury and pain. There are many different types of pain, each with its own psychological qualities (Melzack & Wall, 1988), and each conveying a different type of meaning to the person experiencing the pain. Furthermore, our memory for pain is more complex than one would expect if there were a simple connection between injury and pain (Eich, Rachman, & Lopatka, 1990; Hunter, Philips, & Rachman, 1979). The way in which we record and recall experiences in which pain was experienced varies considerably from person to person, and from occasion to occasion, and is strongly influenced by the emotional and personal significance of the entire event—not merely the site and the extent of the injury. The subject is dealt with in Chapter 3.

Recognition of these serious limitations of the classical theory of pain led Melzack and Wall to formulate their gate control model, which aims to incorporate, or at least allow for, this overwhelming evidence of the complexities of pain.

SUGGESTED READINGS

Melzack, R. (1993). Pain: Past, present and future. *Canadian Journal of Experimental Psychology, 47*, 615–629.

Melzack, R., & Wall, P. (1988). *The challenge of pain.* Harmondsworth, Middlesex, England: Penguin Books.

Wall, P., & Melzack, R. (Eds.). (1989). *Textbook of pain.* NY: Churchill Livingstone.

Weisenberg, M. (1980). Understanding pain phenomena. In S. Rachman (Ed.), *Contributions to medical psychology, Vol. 2* (pp. 79–111). Elmsford, New York: Pergamon Press.

Weisenberg, M. (1987). Psychological intervention for the control of pain. *Behavior Research and Therapy, 25*, 301–312.

CHAPTER 3

Aspects of Pain

MEMORY FOR PAIN

Until recently it was widely believed, based partly on literary observations and psychoanalytic writings, that it is very difficult or impossible to recall one's pain. Research has now shown that, with some interesting exceptions, people are well able to recall their previous pains, and are particularly accurate in doing so if they are given cues to assist the recall process (Hunter, Philips, & Rachman, 1979; Rachman & Eyrl, 1989; Rachman & Philips, 1980; Salovey, Smith, Turk, Jobe, & Willis, in press). They are also capable of recognizing descriptions of their previous episodes of pain.

Complaints of pain, present or past, are the main stimuli for seeking medical help (Dunnell & Cartwright, 1972), and many diagnostic and therapeutic decisions are influenced by the person's recall of his/her pain and its attributes. Indeed the effects of many forms of treatment are still gauged, to some extent, by changes in the patient's report of his or her pain experiences. For these reasons, and because of the growing application of psychological procedures in the treatment of pain, an investigation was undertaken by Hunter, Philips, and Rachman (1979). They assessed the memory for head pain reported after an invasive test procedure by sixteen neurosurgical patients, who were divided into two groups in order to examine the decay of memory over time. One group of patients recalled the pain after an interval of five days and the other group recalled the pain after an interval of one day and then again after five days.

Contrary to expectations, the recall of pain was accurate, and showed little decay over time. The small number of patients who made specific errors when recalling their pain had experienced high levels of pain and emotion at the time of the initial assessment. (See also Lander & Hodgins, 1992; Rachman & Eyrl, 1989; Salovey et al., in press.)

In common with a variety of other psychological states, such as depression, when people are in *pain* their memories of earlier experiences are however influenced by their present state. That is, we are subject to state-dependent memory effects, and as a result our recollections of past episodes of pain tend to be influenced by the state we are in when the recollection takes place. During a period when we are free of pain, we are less likely to recall earlier episodes of pain, or more probably, to recall the earlier episodes of pain as having been less intense than they appeared to be at the time when they actually occurred. On the other hand, if our recollections of earlier episodes of pain are made while we are currently experiencing pain, then we are more likely to recall the earlier episodes as having been as intense or even more painful than they were at the time they actually took place. A full explanation of state-dependent memory for pain remains to be developed, but there is good evidence that these changes in memory are actually mediated, to some extent, by the unpleasant mood which generally is associated with the presence of pain. For example, Eich et al. (1990) studied the menstrual pain experiences of 25 subjects and found that the presence of menstrual pain promoted the retrieval of unpleasant events only when the pain was accompanied by an increase in unpleasant affect. If these results are confirmed, it may mean that recollections of past episodes of pain are likely to be less influenced by mood, and therefore more accurate, if the painful episode is no longer associated with unpleasant affects, or perhaps was never associated with unpleasant affect. Some support for the idea of a state-dependent effect in the memory for pain comes from a study from Bryant (1993), who found that those chronic pain patients who reported increased pain or depression over the course of their study overestimated their memory of the initial pain or depression. Smith and Safer (1993) reported a comparable phenomenon in which overestimations of previous episodes of pain were associated with intense pain and underestimation with reduced pain. The experience of pain comprises at least three major dimensions: sensory, evaluative and affective. Presumably it is the affectively charged memories that are most open to modification or distortion (e.g., Hunter, Philips, & Rachman, 1979). From the clinician's point of view, it is worth bearing in mind that the recollection of affectively loaded memories of pain is more likely to be subject to state-dependent variations than are pain memories that are relatively free of affect.

A vivid and dramatic illustration of the interaction between memory and pain was provided by a remarkable incident that occurred in one of our patients.

While driving her daughter to school one morning the woman's car was struck by another vehicle, causing considerable damage and some injuries. After she, and her daughter, received treatment at the local hospital, they were discharged and went home. The accident was soon followed by the development of severe pain in the lower back that was not responsive to medication and persisted for several months. She commenced psychological treatment of her chronic pain problem and over a period of months made slow but steady progress. Her pain declined in frequency and intensity, but she had almost no recollection of the events immediately prior to, during, and after the motor vehicle accident.

One afternoon, driving to a therapy session, she witnessed a motor vehicle accident involving two other cars. Her own car was not involved on this occasion and sustained no damage other than being struck by a small piece from one of the cars involved in the collision. This produced a clear sound and some sensation of impact. The patient arrived at the clinic looking very pale, agitated, and extremely distressed. She was weeping profusely and reported an intensification of the pain in her lower back. She appeared to be extremely frightened and repeatedly described the sound of the metal striking her own car as if this was more relevant to her than the accident she witnessed. As she began to talk about what she had just witnessed, some details of the *original* motor accident became more accessible for her. She started to report feelings, thoughts, and events that she had not recalled before and certainly never mentioned.

As the patient described and clarified her emotional reactions to the scene she had just witnessed, she gradually became calmer and finally regained her composure, color, and sense of humor. Correspondingly, the intensity of the pain in her lower back diminished and by the end of the session had virtually gone.

The patient said that during the accident which she had just witnessed, she heard screaming and this reminded her of a sound that was very similar to one she had heard during the original accident. She was unsure if these sounds were accurate memories of her own screams, or the screaming she would have liked to have expressed during her original accident. The sound of metal hitting the car also reminded her for the first time of a similar sound which she now recalled from the original accident.

For a period after witnessing the second motor vehicle accident she felt frozen with terror and unable to act, and sat in the driving seat gripping the wheel but unable to propel the car. This led her to recall a similar sense of paralysis and entrapment that she had experienced during the original accident and what she describes as "terror," an emotion which she experienced during both accidents.

When she regained the ability to drive her car after witnessing the second accident, she moved it off to the side of the road and had an overwhelming impulse to telephone her daughter to reassure herself that the child was safe. In fact, she found a telephone and immediately called her daughter. During and after the original accident, the patient was entirely focused on reassuring herself that her daughter was safe and being cared for. She remembers feeling desperate to remain with her daughter but she had been unable to do so in the hospital as the two of them were being treated in separate sections of the emergency room. She now remembered feeling doubly trapped—literally trapped in the car after the accident before being lifted out and taken to hospital, and trapped again when she was unable to gain access to her daughter.

The patient recalled that her overwhelming fear at the time of the original accident was that her daughter might have been severely injured or killed, and as she spoke of it with great anguish, said that she had been terrified that the child would be lost "and everything would be gone for us." She wept when recalling these memories and demonstrated emotions of a severity and urgency that had never been encountered in any of the previous twelve sessions.

Witnessing the second accident appears to have provoked a recollection of many of the details and the accompanying emotion of the original accident, which had previously had not been accessible to her. It also provided a remarkable illustration of how the recollection of an intensely emotional experience contributed to an intensification of the pain, and that when she was finally able to describe the original incident in calm and clear terms, the pain diminished.

Re-Experiencing Pain

Part of the reason for the continuation of the mistaken belief that we are incapable of remembering pain arose from an understandable confusion between the ability to recall a painful experience and the ability to *re-experience* it. There is an important distinction between these two phenomena, and it is easy to demonstrate during seminars or lectures. If you ask people to recall a painful episode from their life they are almost always able to give a reasonably good description of what they felt and thought at the time, for example, "I bumped my elbow against the wall and experienced an immediate sharp pain which then radiated down my forearm. It lasted for 3 minutes." If you then go on to ask the same person to re-experience, to regain the very same pain in their elbow, and to do so at will and on request, they are almost invariably unable to do so. We are able to recall the nature and circumstances of the pain, but unlike our easy ability to re-form a visual experience (e.g., imagine the front of your home), we are rarely able to recreate a previous pain. This inability to re-experience past pains was confused with the ability to recall episodes of pain. We suspect that part of the reason for our difficulty in re-experiencing pain is that it usually involves discomfort or distress, and we therefore have an automatic braking system which prevents us from recreating the pain at will. If that apparent barrier can be suspended, we expect that people will be far more successful in re-experiencing pain voluntarily.

In a recent study of vivid memory for everyday pains Morley (1993) concluded that the memories for these events are "readily retrievable" (p. 55), and at the same time confirmed that the sensory re-experiencing of the pain was not reported by these subjects.

Inaccuracies in recall can be reduced by using standardized instruments such as the McGill Pain Questionnaire, but best of all, patients who are completing a psychological management program are well advised to make daily or even hourly recordings of their levels of pain, thereby circumventing the need to depend on one's memory.

Despite the comparative accuracy of pain recall, there is a tendency for people to overpredict *future* pains.

The Overprediction of Pain

There is a consistent pattern in the way that people predict painful experiences, whether naturally occurring or contrived (Rachman & Arntz, 1991). There is a strong tendency for people to overpredict how much pain they will experience. But these overpredictions of the intensity, and probability, of the pain tend to decrease after people have made an overprediction, and they tend to increase after an *underprediction*. After an episode in which a person experiences significantly more pain than anticipated, there is a strong tendency to make an over overprediction on the next, and following, occasions. One "overcorrects."

However, after making a correct prediction, subsequent predictions tend to be unchanged. Underpredicted episodes of pain are experienced as being more aversive than those that are more correctly predicted or overpredicted.

These patterns of prediction and overprediction resemble the way in which people predict frightening experiences (Rachman & Bichard, 1988). There is a difference however, in that reports of fear tend to decrease with repeated trials, but in the case of pain, repeated exposures to the aversive stimulus are not always followed by habituation. There is converging evidence that underpredicted pain is more aversive than correctly or overpredicted pain of equal intensity: it is experienced as more painful, related to increased levels of fear, and also to escape and avoidance behavior (Alloy & Tabachnik, 1984). It appears that overpredictions of pain persist as long as people continue to attach excessive weight to the occurrences of the painful event and to disregard nonpainful occurrences. Overpredictions of pain can be established quickly, but are slow to decline. Several disconfirmations appear to be required before overpredictions decline, but a single unpredicted painful event may be all that is needed to produce a large increment in the predictions of subsequent distress.

The systematic collection of pain predictions and pain reports provides the basis for a valuable learning experience for patients, enables them to gain improved accuracy, and, importantly, provides them with the sense that they are gaining an improved understanding of the pain and its variations. The personal demonstration of regularity in one's own pain expectations and experiences helps to demystify the experience of pain and offers the promise of increasing personal control over these aversive and distressing events.

The importance of the patients' beliefs about the effects of their behavior on pain is well indicated in a study completed by Waddell and Newton (1993). It was shown that among patients suffering from low back pain, their beliefs about avoidance behavior accounted for 23% of the variance of their disability in daily activities, and 26% of the variance of interference with their working life; even after making allowances for the severity of pain. At least half of the 16 items in the fear-avoidance questionnaire, which was constructed for the purposes of this study, pertain to predictions about the effect of various activities on the occurrence and intensity of anticipated pain. The authors argue that in order "to prevent chronicity, such inappropriate fear-avoidance beliefs would need to be recognized from the acute stage, tackled directly, and changed early before they become fixed" (Waddell & Newton, 1993). And the systematic recording by patients of their predicted pain, followed by the pain actually experienced during the activity, can promote the replacement of the inappropriate beliefs by accurate beliefs.

Overpredictions and underpredictions of pain are classified in a simple manner: The patient is asked to predict, on a 0 to 100 scale, the intensity of the pain that they will experience in a specified situation. This prediction of pain is then compared to the patient's report of the pain that is actually experienced in the specified situation, and the difference between the pain predicted and the pain reported enables one to classify as an overprediction or underprediction. So for example, if a patient predicts that he or she will experience a pain that has the intensity of 80/100 when lifting a heavy weight, and then reports that the pain actually experienced when lifting the weight was only 60/100, this is an overprediction of 20 points, or 25%. Underpredictions are recorded if the reported pain exceeds the predicted pain.

With repeated trials, episodes, or events, there is a strong tendency for the gap between predictions of pain and reports of pain to become increasingly narrow—with repetition, the prediction of pain becomes increasingly accurate.

The overprediction of painful events may be functional, in that it may serve to prevent distress by ensuring that the person avoids situations or circumstances in which pain might be experienced. But this mode of preventing pain is achieved at some cost because avoidance behavior can become excessive, and in extreme cases may lead to immobility or invalidism. Consistent and extensive avoidance of potentially pain-evoking behavior helps to preserve the expectation of future pain. Pain avoidance behavior is a common response but may serve to exacerbate rather than ameliorate the problem (Philips, 1987c). Reduced physical activity may protect one from expected pain but lead to increased physical and psychological distress in the longer term. If people can learn to predict pain experiences with increasing accuracy, as the laboratory evidence indicates, it may provide a safeguard against the development and persistence of serious overpredictions of pain and the unfortunate consequences for the person's behavior.

There is also some evidence that high levels of anxiety promote overpredictions of pain (Rachman & Arntz, 1991). Confirmation of a close functional connection between the prediction of a painful event and fear, and the emergence of avoidance behavior may ultimately open the way for the development of more effective techniques for overcoming unwanted avoidance behavior—by a direct attack on the overpredictive basis of such behavior, preferably combined with attempts to reduce any associated anxiety.

The correction of overpredictions of pain may be of considerable therapeutic value. They probably reduce the tendency to avoidance and provide a platform for the changes in behavior that form a central part of most psychological management programs. In order to assist the patient in achieving greater accuracy in prediction, it is essential to collect information about the person's prediction of pain in particular situations and then to compare these predictions with the reports of the pain that were actually experienced. Most patients are, of course, unaware of their tendency to overpredict the intensity and probability of pain, and it is only by the systematic collection of such information that they and the therapist can be made aware of the occurrence and extent of these overpredictions, and their probable connection to avoidance behavior.

Therapists should also recognize that *underpredictions* of pain are likely to exacerbate the aversiveness of the experience of pain, and may give rise to prolonged and inflated expectations of future pain (Arntz & Peters, 1995); where such underpredictions occur after the therapeutic program has already made some progress, a temporary relapse is not unusual.

Psychogenic Pain

Many of the patients referred to psychological programs have been told directly or implicitly, that their pain is not authentic—it is "merely" psychological.

The concept of psychogenic pain is based on the outdated specificity theory of pain and is misleading. In growing recognition of the inadequacy of the concept, it is gradually fading from use but may yet resurface in a modified form in the newly introduced concept of "somatoform" pain, a term used in DSM IV (APA, 1994).

The central assumption underlying the concept of psychogenic pain is that there is, or should be, a direct, proportional, and temporal relation between an injury or abnormality and pain. Hence, pain reported in the absence of identifiable injury, illness, or dysfunction, is "psychological" in origin. The further implications are that psychological pain is distinct from other experiences of pain, and/or less authentic than other experiences of pain. Disproportionate or untimely reports of pain tend to be regarded as psychogenic. The description of the pain as "psychogenic" is extended to pain reports that are thought to exceed the severity of the injury or illness, and/or reports of pain that emerge some time after the injury was incurred; or pain reports that emerge or persist long after the injury has healed or the illness has passed. However, if the central assumption of a direct, temporal, and proportionate relation between injury and pain is false, then the foundation of the concept of psychogenic pain is removed.

The diagnosis of psychogenic pain by a process of exclusion is insufficient and there is a need for positive evidence to support the concept. In the strict sense, the term *psychogenic pain*, means pain that is *caused* by psychological factors (e.g., "psychological processes may produce pain")

(Merskey, 1980). An example of how the term has been used to infer a causal connection between psychological factors and pain is provided by Blumer and Heilbronn (1982), who argue that ''chronic pain is then the somatic expression of an unresolved psychic pain.'' A broader use of the term was encouraged by Freud's early writings, notably in the case of Elizabeth R., who was said to be ''using her physical feelings (of pain) as a symbol of her mental ones'' (Freud, 1893, p. 144).

However, in practice the term ''psychogenic'' is most often used loosely to refer to the prolongation of pain or the exacerbation of the pain by psychological factors, rather than in the narrow, strictly causal sense. Frequently the term *psychogenic* is used to refer to the occurrence of *behavior* that appears to be inconsistent with, or disproportionate to, the cause of the pain.

Weaknesses in the conception of psychogenic pain should not be allowed to obscure an interesting and important phenomenon, namely that pain reports are often discordant with pain behavior and at times seem to deny anatomy and physiology. As mentioned earlier, in a majority of cases of chronic low back pain it is not possible to identify a proportionate injury, or an underlying injury or abnormality. Moreover, many people who have significant abnormalities of the spinal system, abnormalities widely believed to be the basis of low back pain, report no pain. In attempting to understand the nature of pain abnormalities, it is necessary to start from a recognition that the ''link between injury and pain is highly variable: injury may occur without pain and pain without injury'' (Melzack & Wall, 1988, p. 3).

Somatoform Pain

In the 1986 revision of the DSM, the term ''psychogenic'' was deleted by the editors on the grounds that it was ''stigmatizing'' (Williams & Spitzer, 1982), and was replaced with the term ''idiopathic pain disorder.'' This revised concept was an improvement but remained lodged in the outdated specificity theory of pain. The first part of the definition centered on a ''preoccupation with pain,'' that had continued for at least six months. The second part of the definition stated that idiopathic pain could not be accounted for by organic pathology or physiological dysfunction, and/or the complaint of pain is "grossly in excess of what would be expected from the physical findings." Although this redefinition was a welcome advance on the earlier inferential definitions, it still implied a partial acceptance of the unwarranted assumption or expectation of a close and necessary connection between abnormality/illness and pain. In the latest edition of the DSM (APA, 1994), idiopathic pain disorder has been deleted and is "replaced" in a sense by *pain disorder.*

Pain disorder is classified as one of seven somatoform disorders, which are broadly defined as disorders in which there are physical symptoms that suggest a medical condition but are not fully explained by that condition. *Somatoform pain disorders* are in turn classified into 3 subtypes; (1) pain disorder with psychological factors, (2) pain disorder with psychological and medical factors, and (3) pain disorder associated with a general medical condition, which is "not considered a mental disorder" (p. 458). A diagnosis of pain disorder requires that pain be the major focus of the problem and of sufficient severity to warrant clinical attention (DSM IV). The pain causes significant distress and/or disability. In the first subtype psychological factors are judged to play the major role in "the onset, severity, exacerbation, or maintenance of the pain" (p. 458) and medical conditions play little or no role in the onset or maintenance of the pain. This new definition is an improvement on the outdated concept of psychogenic pain, but lacks specificity.

The second subtype is similar in content but places greater emphasis on the contribution made by the person's medical condition. The third subtype is closely related to a diagnosed medical condition that is not "mental." One regrettable and unnecessary feature of this otherwise progressive change is the retention of the unjustified classification of two of the three pain disorders as types of mental disorders. The first two subtypes of pain disorder, associated with psychological factors and/or medical factors, are included as mental disorders and carefully distinguished from the third type of pain disorder which is said to be not a mental disorder.

Moreover, the new classification lacks specificity. However, it compensates by its implicit recognition of the complex connections between psychological factors and the experience of pain. It also implicitly accepts the fact that instances in which the pain and injury or illness are not concordant are common and indeed an intrinsic feature of many pain experiences. The lack of a close correspondence between a detectable abnormality or injury and the pain should not provide a cause for suspicion. It is in the nature of pain.

Participants in pain-relief programs need to be informed authoritatively, and repeatedly, that pain which occurs and/or persists in the absence of proportionate (or any) detectable injury or illness can be as distressing and disabling as any other type of pain—and is believable and indeed extremely common.

Pain and Depression

Pain and depression are commonly associated (Brown, 1990; Sullivan, Reesor, Mikail, & Fisher, 1992). On the basis of results of population surveys carried out in the United States in recent years, Magni and Caldieron (1990) calculated that 14.4% of the population of the United States between the ages of 25 and 74 suffer from chronic pain to the joints and musculoskeletal system, and that as high as 18% of the population with chronic pain were found to have concurrent depression (in contrast to 8% of the population who do not have chronic pain). Although the figures vary from study to study, the weight of the evidence is clear. Patients with chronic pain problems are two to five times as likely as comparable but pain-free people, to experience depression. For a significant minority the depression is so severe as to earn a diagnosis of a major affective disorder. To take one example, in a detailed study of 100 men suffering from chronic low back pain, Atkinson and Slater (1991) found that after the date of pain onset, the patients had more than nine times the risk of developing major depression than did comparable but pain-free subjects who participated in other epidemiological studies. The overwhelming majority suffered from recurrent episodes of major depression. These results may, however, be somewhat inflated because the patients were drawn from V.A. hospital patients, a group who tend to have a higher rate of psychiatric problems; in addition the patients had an unusually long chronic pain duration, with the mean of greater than 15 years.

The close connection between depression and chronic back pain is illustrated in a study of 37 depressed and 32 nondepressed patients studied by Haythornthwaite, Sieber, and Kearns (1991). On all the important measures of pain (intensity, more extensive pain behavior, greater interference due to pain), the depressed patients obtained higher scores. So, pain patients are prone to depression, and depressed patients are prone to pain. In his study of 243 patients suffering from arthritic pain Brown (1990) also concluded that pain predicts depression.

Depression is associated with a range of other problems, such as anxiety disorders, and it is always difficult to distinguish cause and effect. Are people depressed because of the pain, or is the chronic pain mediated by the depression?

Gamsa (1990) tackled head-on the question of whether emotional disturbance precipitates chronic pain or whether it is more probably a consequence of such pain. She compared 163 sufferers of chronic pain with 81 control subjects on their personal history and on current emotional status, and concluded that overall, ''pain was found to be related to more current depression and less current life satisfaction, but was not associated with most of the personal history variables examined'' (p. 183). ''These results suggest that emotional disturbance in pain patients is more likely to be a consequence than a cause of chronic pain. The dangers of routinely ascribing intractable pain to psychological causations'' (p. 183) are noted. Although the pain patients were at the time of the investigation significantly more depressed than the control group patients, the self-reported lifetime depression of the patients was significantly lower than the self-reported depression of the control patients. Persuasive though her argument is, too great of a dependence on information of this kind that is collected retrospectively, years after the events, is unwarranted. The need for a large-scale prospective study to settle this question is as obvious as it is difficult and expensive to arrange. As far as it goes however, Gamsa's study clearly supports the idea that emotional disturbances, including depression, are more often a consequence than a cause or contributor to chronic pain problems—a view supported by Brown (1990), and Flor, Behle, and Birbaumer (1993), among others. And indeed, it should come as no surprise to learn that persistent pain is depressing.

The clinical significance of associated depression can be considerable. Poor cooperation and drop-outs are common among depressed pain patients (e.g., Sullivan, Reesor, Mikail, & Fisher, 1992), but on the other hand, decreases in pain are followed by decreases in depression. Fortunately, decreases in the depression are likewise followed by declines in pain severity and persistence. There is also a suggestion that chronic pain problems that are accompanied by depression (which usually is cyclical) do not last as long as pain problems unaccompanied by depression (Sullivan & D'Eon, 1990). As Sullivan and colleagues (1992) point out, the tendency to neglect direct treatment of the depression in pain management programs should be corrected. Depression responds moderately well to psychological and/or pharmacological treatment.

SUGGESTED READINGS

Eich, E., Rachman, S. J., & Lopatka, C. (1990). Affect, pain, and autobiographical memory. *Journal of Abnormal Psychology, 99*, 174–178.
Hunter, M., Philips, H. C., & Rachman, S. J. (1979). Memory for pain. *Pain, 6*, 35–46.
Rachman, S. J., & Philips, H. C. (1980). *Psychological and behavioral medicine.* NY: Cambridge University Press.
Salovey, P., Smith, A. F., Turk, D. C., Jobe, J. B., & Willis, G. B. (in press). The accuracy of memory for pain: Not so bad most of the time.

CHAPTER 4

A Cognitive Approach
to the Problem
of Pain

RATIONALE

The cognitive revolution in psychology radically altered clinical work, including the way in which pain is construed and modified. As mentioned earlier, the critical contribution to the psychology of pain was made by Melzack and Wall who recognized the insufficiency of traditional explanations of pain and went on to introduce the gate control model (Melzack & Wall, 1965; Melzack & Wall, 1988). The model incorporates the powerful, often overriding influence of psychological factors in pain experiences, and opened the door to a modern psychology of pain. Although the gate control model cleared the way for a fully psychological theory of pain, the details and mechanisms of this new psychology remain to be elaborated.

The case for introducing cognitive elements into the treatment of pain has been made, among others, by Holzman and Turk (1986) and Turk and Rudy (1992). They note that the cognitive approach developed out of behavior therapy, and hence incorporated the emphasis on operant conditioning, the importance of pain *behavior*, and the role of reinforcers (see especially Fordyce, 1974, 1976). The cognitive approach emphasizes the person's appraisal of and understanding of his or her pain experiences and leads to a wider view of the determinants of pain and its modification. This approach has expanded from the purely behavioral one, and while the importance of behavior remains unchanged, interest is now paid to the cognitions which precede, accompany, and follow the pain experiences.

Turk and Rudy point out that psychological problems in chronic pain can be caused by a variety of factors including: misuse of medication, occupational disability, financial difficulties, prolonged litigation, disruption of social and personal activities. Moreover, the "experience of medical limbo" (1992, p. 103), that is, suffering from a painful condition that defies conventional diagnosis and from which people are led to infer that the causation is psychiatric or an undiagnosed life-threatening disease, is itself a cause of significant stress. What they refer to as the "mysterious" quality of chronic pain (see following paragraphs) can provide the basis for distressing negative cognitions; pain that is irregular, unpredictable, uncontrollable, and difficult for people to understand can easily lead to the general belief that the pain is indeed mysterious. This unhelpful belief often rests on unwarranted assumptions about the precision, range of knowledge, and understanding of modern medicine, and a complementary and specific belief that there *should* be an explanation for one's continuing pain. The absence of a satisfactory and precise medical explanation can, in these circumstances, turn into a source of anxiety about the inexplicability of the problem.

The fundamental assumption of the cognitive approach is expressed by Turk and Rudy: "The cognitive behavioral perspective suggests that behavior and emotions are influenced by interpretations of events, rather than solely by characteristics of the event itself. Thus, pain, when interpreted as signifying ongoing tissue damage or life-threatening illness, is likely to produce considerably more suffering and behavioral dysfunction than it is is viewed as being the result of a minor injury, although the amount of nociceptive input in the two cases may be equivalent" (p. 103). Although pain is generally instigated by injury or illness, psychological factors tend to become more prominent if and when the levels of pain persist and result in, or are associated with, disability. Psychological factors are particularly important in *chronic* pain.

Negative interpretations of one's pain and negative expectations about one's prospects and ability to exert control over pain, are believed to be crucial in the experience of chronic pain. These cognitions are also believed to be crucial in the experience of chronic pain. These cognitions are also believed to have a direct effect on behavior, commonly leading to restricted physical activities and decreasing ability. Given then that the cognitive activity of patients with chronic pain makes a significant contribution to the experience itself and its persistence, consequences, abatement, and modification, the identification of pertinent cognitions, and their therapeutic modification, have become important therapeutic goals (e.g., Jensen, Turner, & Romano, 1994).

COGNITIONS

Pain that is interpreted as signifying a catastrophic illness or serious disability tends to be severe and persistent; pain that is interpreted as benign tends to be milder and limited.

The patient's beliefs about the significance of the pain can be critical. A weakening or removal of irrational beliefs is comforting in its own right and also paves the way for important behavioral gains. These are some of the common beliefs about chronic pain:

- "The presence of pain means that I have an underlying illness or injury." (The common implication is that, unless the underlying injury or illness is identified and dealt with, the pain will continue unrelieved or even get worse.)
- A related and extremely common belief, predating the work of Melzack and Wall, is the idea that all pains are the direct, and proportionate, result of an injury or illness. The implication is that the pain cannot be reduced unless and until the "cause" is identified. "Since there is little or nothing I can do to help myself, pain relief will depend totally on the professional medical care that I receive." This belief, with its implication of helplessness, is a

recipe for passivity. "Nothing can be done until they find the hidden cause."
- Another common belief is that modern medical science can provide explanations and remedies for virtually all symptoms, pains, complaints, illnesses. (A common implication of this belief is that if the medical services cannot find the "true cause" of the pain, that indicates the presence of a rare or serious illness or injury.) This belief also encourages passivity.

The presence of one or another of these beliefs generates a skeptical attitude to the purpose and value of psychological treatment. For example, patients often say something along these lines: "This referral to a psychologist means that my physician regards my pain as nonauthentic in some sense." The referral seems to invalidate the authenticity of the pain, and may call into question the patient's mental stability: "Little or no benefit can be expected from psychological treatment, unless and until the cause of my pain is identified."

The elicitation and full consideration of such beliefs is a vital part of CBT, and methods for assessing these cognitions are described in Chapter 6. Some of the beliefs are extremely common and as the newer view of pain is not widely known, therapists have an important educational role.

The cognitive part of the program proceeds in 8 steps:

1. Provide modern information about the nature of pain.
2. Elicit the patient's pain cognitions.
3. Relate the cognitions to avoidance behavior, pain sensations, passivity/activity.
4. Assemble the patient's evidence for these cognitions.
5. Encourage the patient to consider some alternative explanations for the pain.
6. Assist the patient to assemble evidence to support or disconfirm the alternative explanation.
7. Introduce behavioral exercises and experiments to support or deny the major cognitions.
8. Discuss the nature and implications of the new cognitions.

The cognitions can be elicited in the course of clinical interviews, supplemented by standardized questionnaires (see Chapter 6). Information should also be collected about previous pain and other medical problems, both of the patient and of relatives and friends. The patient's understanding of the pain experience is often found to be strongly influenced by the experiences undergone by people known to the patient. Once the cognitions have been identified and discussed, the therapist encourages the patient to consider the implications of the cognitions. Specific attention should be paid to the relationship between the cognition and the patient's current behavior, especially the avoidance behavior. Similarly, the implication of various bodily sensations or the interpretation for these should be considered. The psychological and behavioral consequences of the cognitions in terms of helplessness, passivity or activity, optimism, and so on, need to be discussed.

ASSEMBLING THE EVIDENCE

After the cognitions have been identified, the therapist assists the patient's assembly of evidence to support or disconfirm the cognitions. At the same time the therapist should attempt to elicit from the patient the kinds of evidence and experiences that he or she would regard as important in evaluating the cognitions—in this way, preparatory material can be gathered for the design of the behavioral experiments to follow.

When the patient's major cognitions and their implications have been fully discussed, the therapist encourages the patient to generate some alternative explanations. So for example, if the patient has a strongly held belief in the idea of a simple and direct connection between pain and an underlying injury, they might also be encouraged to consider the possibility that the relationship between pain and injury is complex, and that there are therefore additional possible interpretations of their own pain experiences. At first, patients tend to find the generation of alternative explanations somewhat difficult but this can be facilitated by the use of the video instructional tape (see page 76) and by discussions within the group. In the group meetings the patients are exposed to the views of fellow sufferers, and learn that it is possible to have more than one potential explanation for experiencing pain. Once they recognize this possibility, the process of generating alternative explanations becomes easier. The group meetings also provide a useful opportunity for the patients to test the structure and rationality of their alternative explanations.

The next step is to help the patient assemble evidence and arguments to support or disconfirm the alternative explanations. This leads naturally into a discussion of behavioral changes, and to the design of specific behavioral exercises. For example, if one of the alternative explanations for the patient's excessive and persistent avoidance of activity is an inflated expectation of the intensity of pain level experienced, a simple set of behavioral tests can be designed. In these the patient predicts the amount of pain that will be experienced in the highly specific set of circumstances, then carries out the relevant activity and reports on the amount of pain actually experienced. Repetitions of these simple behavioral experiments generally lead to a correction of the person's anticipation of pain, making them increasingly accurate, and ultimately enabling them to shed any unnecessary and disabling avoidance behavior.

Collection of fresh and enlightening information should concentrate on a search for regularities and predictability in the pain experience, the patient's gradually increasing control of the pain experience, significant improvements in behavior, reductions in the sense of helplessness, and decreasing depression. This process can be facilitated by the use of "behavioral experiments" which are designed to test particular negative cognitions (e.g., "If I carry out this simple exercise the pain will reach 80/100"). These experiments form an important part of cognitive-behavior therapy (Hawton, Salkovskis, Kirk, & Clark, 1989), and have direct application in pain work.

As the patient begins to make progress, encourage him or her to begin contributing to the design and evaluation of the exercises and to make suggestions for new exercises. An active participation is useful in facilitating treatment and in preparing the patient for a self-help management program to ensure continuity of action. In the closing stages time should be set aside for a discussion of potential problems (e.g., temporary recurrences of pain during periods of stress) and how the patient will deal with them.

In general, the therapist will use all opportunities to bring to the attention of the patients the connections between cognitions and behavior, and how they interrelate. Patients should be encouraged to generate examples of how their cognitions help to determine their behavior, and how changes in behavior begin to modify their cognitions. Here again, discussions within the group can be particularly helpful as patients learn from each other of the reciprocity between behavior and cognitions.

In the cognitive aspects of the program, as in all others, it is essential to collect quantitative data whenever possible. The range and believability of the various cognitions is assessed prior to treatment, mid-course, at the end of treatment, and once again at follow-up. Research on the effects of Cognitive Behavioral Treatment (CBT) as applied to other problems strongly suggests that those patients whose negative and irrational cognitions are subdued by the end of treatment have a much better chance of maintaining their therapeutic improvement after the conclusion of treatment. It is highly probable that a similar relationship exists between the posttreatment cognitions of patients who have completed a pain management program and their long-term progress. The elimination or significant weakening of negative cognitions is of course a good prognostic sign, just as the persistence of strongly believed irrational cognitions at the end of treatment is likely to be a cautionary sign of some recurrent problems, and with that in mind the therapist should make additional efforts to help the patient modify the irrational cognitions.

SUGGESTED READINGS

Hawton, K., Salkovskis, P., Kirk, J., & Clark, D. (Eds.). (1989). *Cognitive behavior therapy for psychiatric problems.* Oxford: Oxford University Press.

Holzman, A., & Turk, D. (Eds.). (1986). *Pain management: A handbook of psychological treatment approaches.* NY: Pergamon Press.

Jensen, M. P., Turner, J. A., & Romano, J. M. (1994). *Journal of Consulting and Clinical Psychology, 62,* 172–179.

Pearce, S. (1983). A review of cognitive/behavioral methods for the treatment of chronic pain. *Journal of Psychosomatic Research, 27*(5), 431–440.

Turk, D. C., & Rudy, T. E. (1992). Cognitive factors and persistent pain: A glimpse into Pandora's box. *Cognitive Therapy and Research, 16,* 99–122.

CHAPTER 5

Characteristics of the Training Program

DEFINITION OF THE PROGRAM

Referrals are received and evaluated, and patients are treated by psychologists, utilizing pharmacists, physical therapists, and physicians as consultants in the selection and management of exercises, and of drug reduction. It is a highly structured, time-limited program designed to produce its initial effects over a 9-week period. Nine discrete pain management strategies are delineated and practiced during the weekly sessions, so that patients gradually develop a competence in the management of their chronic pain problems.

It has been structured to allow the treatment of patients in groups, as this is cost-effective and provides benefits not easily provided by treatment sessions. Each group member learns that there are considerable individual differences in the potency and utility of the techniques taught, reinforcing the need for each person to develop his or her own methods. It provides support, vicarious instruction, and encouragement to the participants.

In addition, and of great importance, is the inhibition of discussion of irrelevant material and of complaints per se. Pain patients are rarely interested in each other's complaints and this acts as an important social constraint on the continuation of maladaptive talk. Finally, participation in a group can break the isolation that many of these patients feel, bringing them into contact with other people in a social setting. Many have reported that they gain a sense of proportion with respect to their own problems by seeing the dilemmas and distress suffered by others with similar problems.

Despite the benefits of group work, individual sessions are recommended for people whose social anxiety would inhibit their participation in a group, or those who have other pressing problems likely to disrupt the progress of the group. For these people, more treatment time may be necessary to allow a longer focus on certain aspects of their problem (e.g., depressive reaction).

An outpatient treatment protocol has been chosen because it allows the participants to practice strategies and methods of management in their own environment. With the aim of returning the person to as close an approximation of a normal and fulfilling life as possible, this type of practice is crucial. Generalization of skills is facilitated, specific problems that arise (with respect to spouse or partner reactions, work difficulties, exercise constraints) can be dealt with as they occur, and the evolution of more appropriate strategies for that person can be encouraged. Time between sessions is an important ingredient of the method (recommended length is approximately one week). This allows time for the person to practice the new skills and deal with the impact of a new technique on his or her former life patterns.

Many of the techniques presented can be modified for use in an inpatient setting, but the manual has been designed specifically to provide an outpatient program and does not cover some of the intricacies of inpatient work.

SETTING FOR TREATMENT AND CROSS-DISCIPLINARY INVOLVEMENT

The current program can be undertaken by the psychologist within a multidisciplinary clinic or by a cognitive-behavioral clinician within a psychology department or private practice, drawing on the consultative expertise of physician, pharmacist, and physiotherapist. The treatment itself is psychological and does not depend on physical techniques such as Transcutaneous Nerve Stimulation (TNS), acupuncture manipulation, or drugs. This setting for treatment is innovative. Most pain clinics are administered by physicians who engage psychologists, full-time or part-time sessionally, to fulfill their psychological function if and when it is deemed suitable. Moving away from the multidisciplinary setting makes it important for the psychologist to establish proper consultative relationships with medical personnel. These are essential for selection and useful in facilitating two ingredients of the program (i.e., graded reduction of analgesics and graded increase in exercise). As long as a cooperative relationship is established with the other specialists, there is no need for a psychologist to be attached to a multidisciplinary pain clinic in order to undertake chronic pain management. Because of the novelty of this nonmedical setting for undertaking chronic pain management, Figure 5.1 illustrates the organization of a chronic pain management service directed from a psychology unit. Although it is not necessary for consultants to work in the same establishment, smooth and regular consultative links are invaluable for efficient treatment.

Physician

It is essential not to select people who would be more appropriately treated by standard medical procedures. This decision cannot be made entirely by the psychologist, but requires the expertise of a physician to assess the results of previous physical evaluations and/or their adequacy (e.g., recency, comprehensiveness). If a physician is not available to work on a sessional basis with the psychologist, it is possible to coordinate in such a way that the relevant specialists' reports are evaluated by the general practitioner. When making the referral, the general practitioner can then evaluate and interpret the physical tests that have been undertaken. It is, however, recommended that a physician with expertise in some area of physical pain be encouraged to join the psychologist on a regular basis in evaluating prospective candidates. This safeguard allows the psychologist to feel more confident when working with some of the complex cases that will be referred. Hesitations on the psychologist's part with respect to the adequacy of the physical evaluation are quickly detected by patients,

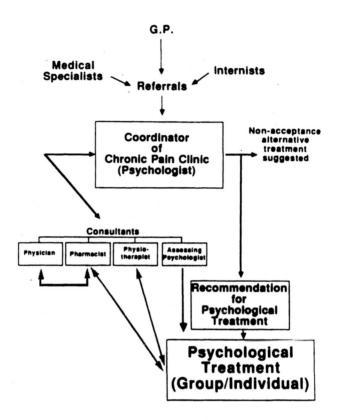

FIGURE 5.1 Organization of psychologically directed pain management service.

who tend to seek repeated reassurance from the medical world that no more sinister cause is operative.

All physical examinations, evaluations, and consultations must be done *prior* to the onset of any treatment so that the patient has no reason to refrain from involvement in the program. It is wise to delay the onset of treatment until these evaluations have been completed and the physician or consultant is satisfied that the person is an appropriate candidate for psychological management. It is not advisable for any clinical psychologist to treat without this safeguard.

Pharmacist

A large proportion of problem cases referred by GPs and specialists are people with serious drug dependencies. In fact, one of the most likely reasons for referral to a psychological service is the recognition by referring physicians of escalating drug dependency problems that are drawing them into overprescribing. Many patients themselves describe their pain problem as rivaled only by their dependency on drugs and their side-effects. Pharmacists can help identify the small percentage of cases in whom drug dependency problems have become sufficiently serious to necessitate detoxification prior to the onset of pain management. The experience of a pharmacist is useful in judging the suitability of candidates for an outpatient program, given their level of dependency. In addition, an independent judgment of the extent of primary drug abuse is useful. Such patients are rarely seen in pain management services that make clear at the onset to both referring physician and patient that the program entails a graded reduction in drugs. However, it is possible to come across this type of patient, and they are not suitable for a self-management approach.

For these reasons it is unwise for psychologists to undertake chronic pain management without the consultative advice of a pharmacist. Such a specialist can help not only with the selection of cases suitable for psychological management, but also formulate a drug profile for each person, making recommendations for a graded reduction regime. In addition, the pharmacist will need to coordinate with a physician so that progressive reductions of drugs can be undertaken, following the graded reduction program. Different methods can be used. Some centers (e.g., the University of Washington Pain Clinic) use a pain cocktail method. This cocktail often consists of three major components:

1. a long-acting oral effective narcotic analgesic (usually methadone);
2. a long-acting oral effective sedative (phenobarbitol); and
3. a taste or flavor-masking device (cherry syrup, Maalox, etc.).

These may be enhanced by other ingredients, such as acetaminophen (analgesic), hydroxyzine (sedative), and fedux (flavor-masking agent).

Alternatively, the graded reduction or deconditioning (as opposed to detoxification) can be undertaken using a liquid equivalent to the drug currently being used by the patient, mixed with a flavor base. This ensures an exact equivalent between the drugs used by the person before entering the program.

Needless to say, the composition of the liquid equivalent needs to be carefully considered by a trained pharmacist, preferably one with knowledge of chronic pain management. If it is not possible for the psychologist to coordinate with a specific pharmacist (as is possible within a hospital environment), the GP responsible for the patient may be persuaded to obtain this type of expertise from a local community pharmacist and to write the necessary prescription.

It is difficult to undertake a graded reduction of medications without a liquid equivalent. Tablets are hard to break into equal parts, and capsules make the gradual reduction impossible. In addition, the psychological effect of seeing diminishing amounts of drugs is usefully counteracted by the liquid solution. It allows the person to take the *same amount* of liquid throughout the graded reduction program while the proportion of the drug suspended in the flavoring is reduced. Psychologists are advised not to undertake the management of cases with complex dependency problems if they do not have the help of a pharmacist; they should restrict their chronic pain management work to those patients whose dependency problem is not sufficiently severe to warrant a graded liquid reduction method. An example of a graded reduction program using a liquid equivalent is provided in Appendix I.

Physical Therapist

The involvement of physical therapists is highly desirable. They can provide an assessment of physical fitness of a person that highlights the muscle loss which needs to be remedied by a physical exercise program. They can provide useful advice to the psychologist about how and at what rate to progress toward strengthening the muscle groups. For those unable to obtain physical therapy consultations, most if not all chronic pain patients can benefit from a program of brisk exercise of their choice (walking, swimming, or bicycling). Working from patients' own monitored onset levels of exercise, graded increases in their capacity can be organized and often prove sufficiently efficacious. With a physical therapist's help, specific exercises and stretches can be given to a patient, although the added effects of an individually tailored exercise program have not yet been demonstrated. It is clear that patients appreciate the personal physical therapy assessment and respond more enthusiastically to exercise programs generated for them in this way. If physical therapy consultations are not available, recommend exercises that do not need personal assessment by a physical therapist. These are provided in Appendix II.

If it is possible for the psychologist to coordinate with a local physical therapist, a physical therapy program can be set up and coordinated with the 9-week treatment program. However, the ideas of gradual increase in exercise quotas, setting the onset of the exercise level well below the patient's physical capability, and of making small increments may be novel to the physical therapist and will need to be discussed.

In summary, psychologists can promote an exercise program outside a formal multidisciplinary clinic as long as they remain aware of the importance of:

1. not undertaking treatment of patients for whom a standard medical approach is more appropriate;
2. not undertaking the reduction of complex drug problems without the advice of a pharmacist; and
3. coordinating with a physical therapist if personally tailored exercise programs are needed.

The organization of this psychologically directed pain management approach entails that the direction and treatment be undertaken by the psychologist, but with an important proviso. Advice should be obtained from the appropriate specialists with respect to physical fitness, drug use, and medical issues. The link between the psychologist and the consultants need not be formalized in an established pain clinic and can be organized with GP and local hospital services accordingly. Needless to say, the easier the communication links, the more efficient the treatment program. Best of all, these pain management programs should be provided by an established pain clinic staffed by the necessary team of specialists.

LENGTH OF TREATMENT

From the onset, let patients know the length of time they will be in treatment, and working towards the goals they have set. Nine sessions are the minimum treatment length required to cover the full program. The addition of the 2-week self-monitoring pretreatment period and the posttreatment evaluation (1 week posttreatment), amounts to a 3-month (or a 12-week) period, from start to finish of the program. Emphasizing this to patients at onset encourages them to recognize the need for involvement immediately and continuously during the program. Each session lasts 1 1/2 hours. With a group size of four to seven people, this is sufficient time, as long as the therapist keeps within the suggested sessional structure. Explain to the patients in the group the time limitations of the sessions, to avoid resentment of the structure. For individual treatment sessions, 1-hour sessions are sufficient.

SUPPORTIVE WRITTEN MATERIAL

It is useful to have supporting written material for patients that reviews the subject discussed in each of the sessions. The patients gradually build up a set of readings that cover the 9-week treatment period and that can be referred to during and after treatment. This is useful to them in a number of ways.

1. Since some of the material will not have been absorbed during the 1 1/2 hour period, it allows them time to absorb it slowly over the next week.
2. It allows them to communicate the content of the treatment to spouse or partner.
3. The materials can be actively used in cases of partial relapse or during problem periods after treatment finishes. It has been found that patients will refer back to their readings and, on some occasions, put themselves through sections of the 9-week package again, in order to remind themselves of techniques they have learned.
4. Finally, because of the mosaic method of presenting material to patients, the sessions interrelate and overlap in many ways. Patients can benefit enormously from rereading some modules in conjunction with others. In particular, the first session, which deals with the orientation of the program and the model of chronic

pain, becomes a valuable foundation to refer back to, while integrating each of the subsequent sessions. In the final session, in which a summary is made for the patient as to how the different sessional materials fit together into one complete jigsaw picture or mosaic, he or she may well wish to refer back to other sessional material.

An example of supportive material for the first session is given in Appendix III. (A full set of sessional handouts can be ordered separately from the Springer Publishing Company in a manual format.) In addition to didactic material, sheets to systematize self-monitoring or homework tasks are useful. They improve adherence and allow the therapist to scan quickly at the onset of the session to see the degree of practice that has been undertaken by each member of the group. Some self-monitoring sheets are recorded by the patient throughout the program (e.g., their exercise regime), while others are completed as a preparation at the onset of the session asking patients to summarize out loud their conclusions from their self-monitoring sheets. This is a useful method for encouraging each patient to monitor their progress and draw conclusions about the problem being monitored (e.g., amount of verbal complaint, utility of specific strategy). Therapist aids for keeping a record of patient problems and compliance of person patients are provided in Appendix IV.

STRUCTURE OF SESSIONS

Each of the nine successive sessions has been planned to cover a different aspect of the problem of chronic pain. In focusing on the effects of such factors as overuse of drugs, inactivity, anxiety, depression, anticipatory avoidance, somatic focusing, and so forth, as well as on explaining the negative effects of many of these factors on pain levels, the session introduces a related technique or strategy that patients can use to counteract the influence of, and thus modulate and reduce, pain. For example, in the session that discusses the effects of inactivity and physical weakness (Session #3), both the practical strategy discussed and the homework assignment relate to increasing activity levels and exercise. In the discussion of depression and depressive reactions to pain episodes (Session #7), the strategy emphasized is that of positive self-talk, entailing the use of a coping statement followed by a coping action.

Although each session is separable, the interlinking of the sessions is clear, and wherever possible the therapist draws this to the attention of the group (e.g., depressive preoccupations with sensation and the effect of somatic focusing upon pain experience [Sessions #6 and 7]). The concept of building a jigsaw puzzle, or amassing the pieces of a mosaic, is useful in encouraging patients to see the necessity of attendance and involvement in each session to get a full picture of their own pain problems and how to manage them. The overall orientation (Session #1) may become evident to some patients only when they reach the end of the 2-month period. However, giving them this overall framework is effective, acceptable, and understandable to chronic pain patients from the outset.

The within-session structure is retained in every session. Sessions begin with a discussion of the homework assignment from the previous week. In Session #1, the assignment to complete the goal sheet is given to patients at their final assessment interview. But in all other sessions, the homework consists of practicing a new tactic or the monitoring of a new factor in preparation for its discussion at the next session. After discussion of homework, a short didactic presentation is made by the therapist. Although patient interruption and discussion is never restricted, encourage patients to sit for a short period of time and listen to some material, giving their reactions at the end. Wherever possible, use specific examples drawn from facts known about members of the group. This method will draw them into the discussion and help them recognize the applicability of the didactic presentation to their own problems. For example, in discussing the role of muscle tension, a particular person's tendency to tighten up shoulders or grind teeth can be used as an example of the kind of bracing and tensing response that can develop among chronic pain patients. Using specific case examples entails the therapist's being adequately acquainted with each patient's problem and the focus that is particularly important for them (see Appendix IV, Therapist Aids). If the therapist undertakes the assessment interview for members of the group (or person treatment), this task is made easy. If this is not the case, the therapist needs to become knowledgeable about each patient, reading carefully the report of the assessing psychologist. (The Therapist Summary Sheet in Appendix IV is a useful reminder during treatment sessions.)

The third section of each session entails demonstration and practice by patients of a strategy specifically related to the didactic discussion. For example, when discussing attention focus and distraction techniques, the immediate effects of focusing on pain, as opposed to external sounds, is demonstrated (Session #6). This is followed by the practice of distraction techniques with relaxation over a 20-minute period.

Finally, specific homework tasks are assigned, utilizing the tactics suggested. Discuss any problems that the group members predict they may have in using the tactic during the next week. Trouble-shooting in this way is a very useful way of circumventing the development of practical problems that will slow up treatment application and reduce compliance. Sometimes a self-monitoring task is suggested in order to prepare the way for the didactic presentation in the next session. For example, patients might be asked to monitor, in their diaries, the stressful stimuli that they notice are associated with peaks in their pain rating. This monitoring of stress and high arousal levels precedes the discussion of the role of the emotional state in pain (Session #5). At the completion of the session, patients collect the self-monitoring forms and supportive material concerning the key concepts dealt with during the session, so that they may review them at home.

The benefit of having this 4-stage structure to the sessions is that it helps the therapist cover a great deal of material in the 1 1/2 hours. It also gives patients the correct expectation about when open discussion is feasible and useful, and when they need to sit back and try to absorb new material.

TACTICS

Types of Tactics

Various methods of dealing with the pain are introduced to the patients over the 9-week treatment program. These methods or tactics are summarized here:

Tactic 1: Relaxation (Session #2)

The reflexive tensing response to pain, which has beneficial effects with acute injury, becomes counterproductive as pain persists. Most chronic pain patients find themselves unable to relax the locus of the pain problem and may subsequently develop habitually raised muscular tension in these areas or may tighten certain muscle groups in response to pain episodes. The capacity to relax the muscles at will is an important self-control technique usefully taught to chronic pain patients. It is included in almost all multidisciplinary pain clinics and is one of the first therapeutic interventions undertaken by psychologists. Philips (1987a) demonstrated that specific effects of relaxation on pain level can be produced within one session. This type of control over both the sensory and affective components of the pain experience is an important demonstration to the patients of the extent to which they can modulate pain levels and bring them under their own control.

Tactic 2: Increasing Activity/Fitness (Session #3)

Many chronic pain patients evolve ways of living with pain that limit their activity and ultimately reduce their fitness. Automatic avoidance of many types of interaction and stimulation takes place (Philips & Jahanshahi, 1985; Zarkowska & Philips, 1985). Patients tend to develop inactive lives not only because of the level of pain that they are experiencing, but also because of their predictions of the effects of activity on subsequent pain levels. This anticipatory avoidance may well be an important ingredient in the disability that develops (Philips & Jahanshahi, 1985). In addition, a disuse syndrome evolves because of the failure to use the body part where the pain occurs. They grow physically weak, unfit, and fatigue easily. Thus, it is important to encourage patients to return to more normal levels of activity tolerance and to increase their stamina for physical activities. It seems likely that while undergoing such activity programs, conditioned avoidance is gradually extinguished.

Tactic 3: Independence from Drugs (Session #4)

The problems of chronic pain patients are a testament to the fact that drugs suitable for acute pain episodes become progressively weaker in the management of chronic pain. Many patients develop dependencies on these drugs and experience associated side-effects (constipation, gastric problems, decreased concentration, mood disturbances). However, the capacity to survive *without* the use of these drugs has to be demonstrated to the patients. It is most easily undertaken if patients perceive drug elimination as a positive step.

Tactic 4: Diffusing/Reducing Emotional Overreactivity (Session #5)

It is commonly reported by pain patients that if they get upset, particularly about pain, the experience intensifies. It is, therefore, useful to teach them specific methods of reducing their autonomic arousal in the face of stressful stimuli. Often they cannot remove these aggravations from their lives, but they can learn different methods of handling them when they occur. The tactic taught in this treatment program is derived from those evolved in the management of anxiety problems, where it has been found to be a potent treatment intervention (Wilson, 1984).

Tactic 5: External Focusing (Distraction) (Session #6)

The focus of attention affects the amount of awareness a person has of a stimulus. It is, therefore, possible for pain patients to shift and manipulate their focus of attention in their own favor, minimizing pain experience and increasing tolerance. This is a cognitive technique, useful in dealing with short, difficult episodes of pain (Turk, Meichenbaum, & Genest, 1983).

Scientific research concurs with common sense in concluding that distraction is a useful method for reducing pain. McCaul and Mallot (1984, pp. 516–533) summarized the main findings on the effects of distraction in this way. Deliberate distraction is capable of reducing pain and distress, and does so more effectively than incidental occurrences of distraction. Secondly, distraction techniques "that require more intentional capacity will be more effective" (p. 516). Thirdly, distraction has more powerful effects on low intensity pain than it does on high intensity pain.

In many circumstances, it is useful to think of the relationship between distraction and pain as a type of balance, in which an increase in pain may make it more difficult to distract oneself, and on the other side, distraction techniques that absorb a lot of attentional capacity will help to submerge the pain. There are, of course, individual differences in the ability to recruit and use distraction techniques, with some patients rapidly acquiring effective skills but others finding it difficult to accomplish. It is possible to improve one's ability to use distraction techniques after specific training, and there is no reason to suppose that any particular patient is inherently incapable of acquiring at lease some skill in the use of distraction techniques.

Tactic 6: Assertion (Session #6)

Chronic pain patients sometimes use complaining about pain and disability, and demonstrating pain, in order to achieve other goals. For example, complaining of pain may act as an indirect method of avoiding housework or a visit to relations. Increasing assertiveness and clarification of the purpose of the complaint will lead to a reduction of this consequence of prolonged pain. Approaching the issue of complaint and conversation about pain in this manner is acceptable to chronic pain patients and leads to much more fruitful consequences than discussions of ''secondary gain.''

Tactic 7: Reappraisal of Pain (Session #7)

An increasing number of techniques are becoming available to patients for modulating pain levels by using thinking, or cognitive, tactics. These techniques can be used on their own or in combination, and patients are encouraged to develop their own techniques, elaborating these reappraisal approaches in their own ways. Some examples of the cognitive tactics taught are redefinition, denial, relocation, and so forth.

Tactic 8: Activity Pacing and Nonavoidance (Session #8)

This tactic represents a culmination of much of the previous work done throughout treatment. It is a general tactic that is made possible because of the patients' use of many other tactics. They are requested to continue work despite pain, using the techniques they have learned to enable themselves to do so. In addition, the whole issue of *pacing* is highlighted, as it allows completion of an activity that had previously seemed impossible. Gradual steps toward a larger goal are efficacious and this is proved to patients over the weeks (e.g., exercise programs).

Tactic 9: Cue-Controlled Relaxation (Session #8)

This method of relaxation has been developed in order to allow patients to induce relaxation within a 3- to 4-minute period, cueing themselves with a word or image that they have previously associated with the longer 20-minute induction process. They can only undertake this method when they have become skilled in the relaxation technique by having practiced for a number of weeks the general relaxation method introduced in Session #2. It is possible to teach this abbreviated version, once the skill is well developed. Patients appear able to invoke this cue method at times when they notice themselves tensing up or when they anticipate that pain may be produced if they continue an activity. It becomes a potent tactic for them, allowing them to pace activities; preventing them from withdrawing and avoiding activities.

Timing of Tactics

From the very beginning of training, it is emphasized to patients that research into chronic pain management is not yet sophisticated enough to predict which particular tactics will suit which patients. We are unable to precisely match techniques with patients, but some techniques have wide value (e.g., relaxation). It is, therefore, up to patients to sample as many methods of managing pain as can be presented to them in the 9 weeks and to select those methods that suit them. This "smorgasbord approach" encourages patients from the start of the program to decide on how they will manage their pain. It is also an important step toward the reduction of the passive invalid role that many of them demonstrate at the onset of treatment, and its replacement by active, coping tactics and attitudes.

The order of presentation of tactics suggested earlier has been found particularly useful for the following reasons. The first three tactics are readily acceptable to patients with chronic pain problems who, at the onset of treatment, will be relying upon a traditional medical model of pain. By the time they reach Session #4, they are much more likely to listen with attention to a discussion of the influence of psychological factors (emotional reactions, attention focus), especially as they will have had three weeks of self-monitoring of their own pain reactions. By the time they reach Sessions #5 and #6, they will have absorbed a great deal of the significance of the Gate Control Model and will work much more readily on cognitive strategies and the modification of emotional reactions.

The issue of reappraisal of pain, if introduced as Tactic #7 (i.e., in week 7), will be an understandable approach that, if undertaken earlier, would have met with lack of comprehension and uncooperativeness. Tactic #8 (activity pacing and nonavoidance) is handled throughout treatment in various ways, although it is not formalized into an approach to pain management until the very end of treatment, when the utility of nonavoidance has been demonstrated to patients week by week. At this time, the majority of patients will have met their physical therapy goal with respect to physical exercise and will have achieved many of the goals they have set with respect to their social, leisure, work, and personal life. In addition, they will have found out, from their own self-monitoring, some of the consequences of overactivity and nonpacing. Dealing with the issue of pacing at this stage allows the therapist to integrate many of the conclusions patients will have drawn during treatment with the evident progress they have made in many areas. Tactic #9 can, of course, only be undertaken when relaxation can be quickly induced, after many weeks of practice, and thus is included near the very end of treatment.

Some tactics take much longer to learn than others and entail repeated weekly reminders and advice from the therapist. An example of this is the gradual learning of progressive muscle relaxation techniques. In addition, the slow reduction of the use of analgesics needs as many weeks as possible. These tactics are, therefore, introduced at the beginning of the program. Gaining compliance in an exercise routine and bringing their exercise capacity to an appropriate level is best undertaken week by week, for as long a period as possible. Exercise is, therefore, introduced early on in the program. Some tactics can be explained and encouraged in one session. If there are a number of different aspects to a method, it may be included in two sessions (e.g., Tactic #5 which is discussed in both Sessions #4 and #6). Some tactics with many aspects can be introduced quickly in one session (e.g., reappraisal strategies entail many possible methods, and these can all be explored in one session). In summary, the ordering of sessions has been determined by several factors. The number of occasions in which the tactics need to be practiced and discussed is relevant. In addition, those tactics that are more difficult for chronic pain patients to accept as important are introduced later in the program, when the Gate Control Model is well established.

A distinction can be made between techniques used for preventive purposes and those used to increase episodic control over pain level. In practice, this distinction may prove somewhat arbitrary, with patients reporting that sequential management of each pain episode leads to prevention (and vice versa, that preventive techniques make episodes less likely). Despite the overlap, the presentation of techniques in terms of the preventive and/or episodic focus is useful to patients and leads them to have the correct expectations about the effect of a strategy on pain levels. This will prevent disappointment and discouragement. For example, in the early stages of learning relaxation, patients should be encouraged to think of it as a preventive strategy or as a long-term insurance against the development of muscular tensing or bracing, which may exacerbate pain. As their skill improves, the specific episodic control that can be achieved using these methods (cue-control strategy) can then be highlighted.

CHAPTER 6

Selection, Assessment, and Preparation for Treatment

SELECTION AND ASSESSMENT

From the outset, it is advisable to set precise selection criteria. In the early stages, newly established therapeutic resources receive a disproportionate number of inappropriate referrals, and the availability of clear criteria is a useful safeguard. The following guidelines can be used to guide the psychologist and other specialists, referring agents, and agencies, and potential patients.

Inclusionary Criteria

There are seven inclusionary criteria:

1. Chronic (more than 6 months duration) and incapacitating pain.
2. Marked reduction in normal daily activities and reduced physical activity. (A "holding" pattern is characteristic of pain patients

awaiting pain cessation. This is characterized by high avoidance patterns, long periods of resting or sleep during the day, and cessation of involvement in leisure activities.)

3. High emotional responses to pain experience. (These can be inferred from the large affective component of the pain experience, increased anxiety in the face of pain, autonomic signs of anxiety associated with pain episodes, night visits to emergency rooms.)

4. Mild to moderate depression. (It is unwise to take on people with severe depression for group sessions if the modification of depression is the focal issue. However, patients with mild to moderate depression, without suicidal risk, respond well to pain management, especially when the depression appears to be significantly exacerbated by pain experience and its consequences.)

5. Environmental gains for pain avoidance and pain behavior (reduced activity and increased complaint).

6. Lack of specific coping strategies to deal with pain experience and the pain problem per se.

7. Evidence of negative cognitions, notably catastrophizing and expressions of helplessness.

Exclusionary Criteria

The seven exclusionary criteria are:

1. People who are involved in unresolved compensation cases or disputes with respect to disability pay, or who are planning and organizing litigation. Although there is controversial evidence on this point, it seems likely that an accurate account of the pain problem, as well as full motivation to make changes, will be undermined under these circumstances. There are indications that people involved in litigation do not make gains in behavioral programs until the litigation is resolved (Derebury & Tullis, 1983; Trief & Stein, 1985), but the evidence is not consistent.

2. Patients for whom alternative effective physical treatments can be provided or who have been inadequately assessed.

3. The fewer the preceding surgical operations they have undergone, the more likely they are to make dramatic changes in their pain

problems. Each additional operation produces its own iatrogenic consequences (scar tissue, etc.), and the pain management program is likely to produce less improvement in people who have had multiple operations. In addition, it is important to encourage referring sources to seek psychological help for the management of chronic pain problems prior to surgery whenever possible. Accepting only those people who have had one or no operations encourages earlier referral by physicians. Psychological management of a problem can eliminate the need for an operation (see Chapter 16, Case #6).

4. Patients whose pain is due to cancer have not been included in this program to date because of their special needs. (However, the program is potentially modifiable for this patient group—see Turk & Rudy 1987.)

5. Patients who are suffering from active psychosis; who have inadequate English comprehension; or have any condition that prevents active and intelligent participation, should not be included.

6. For headache patients, it is advisable to treat female patients following the withdrawal of contraceptive medication, which can produce headaches as a side-effect.

7. Patients who are primary drug abusers are inappropriate candidates for this outpatient treatment program; they are likely to select themselves out when the nature of the program is made clear to them.

INFORMATION FROM REFERRAL SOURCES

In order to make a final decision with respect to suitability, information is gathered from three sources: the referral source, a structured interview with the patient, and from the consultants to the program. This process is shown in Figure 6.1. The first source of information comes from the referring physician, who will be able to provide past consultation reports, a summary of management to date (its form, scope, and effect), and any other information that has been collected over preceding years. If the physician is cognizant of the nature of a psychological program, she or

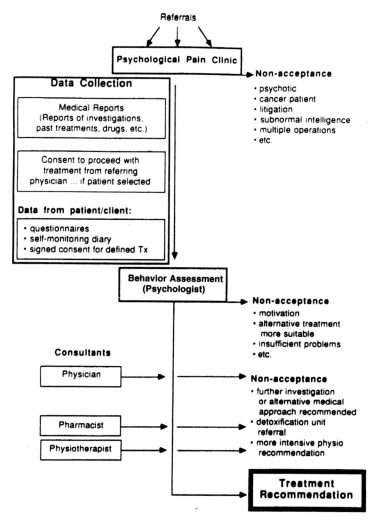

FIGURE 6.1 Information obtained from various referral sources.

he will provide the needed information. As misunderstandings about the nature of psychological intervention are common in the professions and among potential patients, information must be supplied to the referral sources, and hand-outs for patients provided.

STRUCTURED INTERVIEW

The most important component of the assessment procedure is the structured interview with the patient. Within one to two hours, a structured approach can provide the psychologist with information vital to making a judgment about the suitability of the person for a psychological program. Having a structured format allows the interviewer to ensure that all the relevant areas are covered and to focus the discussion. Indeed, the very involvement of patients in this structured assessment can become the first stage of treatment. Their attention is drawn by the questions to particular aspects of the problem, to the interrelationship of variables, to their own lack of coping techniques or goals, the absence of pleasurable activities, and the failure of previous interventions. Although the interview was constructed in order to aid selection, it also provides an excellent opportunity to prepare patients for an active self-management treatment program.

The form of the structured interview is provided in Appendix V. The order of items is designed to allow patients to discuss more complex factors with the knowledge that their basic problems have been understood. The first issue dealt with in this structured interview is the problem as it is perceived by the patient (its characteristics, pattern and course, locus). It has been found that this preliminary discussion allows patients to demonstrate the validity of their pain experience to the interviewer and reduces later reluctance to discuss emotional interactive factors.

The interview continues with an elaboration of associated symptoms, some of which are important in delineating the degree of impairment, while others help the psychologist to evaluate the degree of emotional reaction during pain episodes. This is aided by the clarification of factors that, from the patient's point of view, affect the tolerance of pain. The issue of ''triggers'' is not focused upon, unless raised by the patient. Rather, he or she is asked to delineate *to what extent* any situations or emotional states affect his or her tolerance of pain (i.e., reducing or increasing pain). The aim is not to find *a* cause, but to look at the situational or psychological factors that can influence pain levels.

Inquiring in this manner will also lead to useful information concerning family interactions (the effect of quarrels, emotional times, anger), sexual adjustment (the question of the effect of pain on sex), and activity levels (the effect of pain on vacations and pleasurable activities). This information is usefully related to the Sickness Impact Profile (Appendix VI) to give the assessor an impression of the impact of pain upon the person's marital, sexual, and family relations.

The degree to which the pain problem is interrupting or interfering with the patient's normal life is evaluated in the section of the interview entitled "Consequences." The aim of the interviewer is to get patients to consider how pervasive a problem their pain has become in terms of its interference with normal activity. During this assessment, it is important to establish the prepain level of functioning, especially with respect to physical exercise and social life, in order to estimate the full degree of effects of the problem. Patients may speak of being *unable* to undertake sports activities. Inquiry may prove this due to disinterest, lack of drive, and so forth, rather than simple avoidance of pain.

Finally, an important consequence of persistent pain is the development of dependency on one or more drugs. A clear delineation of current medication use is essential. When this is undertaken, it is often possible to gain a good medication history and to hear of the reasons for shifting medications. Estimates of the likelihood adherence to a new regime can be formulated. An assessment of the attitude to drugs can often be completed after listening to patients' descriptions of drug use. It is quite common to find a negative attitude toward drugs both in terms of attitudes toward their use and their efficacy and yet to find the person trapped into persistent use. It is also important to discover the extent to which they are aware of the side effects of the drugs (at the level being used) and to see what understanding they may have of the mechanisms of operation of their drugs.

After discussion of prescribed and nonprescribed drugs for pain, an inquiry follows about the use of alcohol for the control of pain. Clarify whether there is any current or past alcohol abuse. Where appropriate, the history and current use of other psychoactive drugs should be clarified (amphetamines, marijuana, cocaine).

It is an easy step to move from the discussion of current medication use to a discussion of previous treatment and specialist advice. The methods patients have found to cope with pain (other than drugs) should also be clarified. An incidental effect of such an inquiry (into coping strategies) is that it lays the foundation for the introduction of a self-management approach to pain, with its stress on the development of active coping skills. The patient's attention may be drawn to his or her lack of strategies or defenses against pain by the question itself.

The patients' explanations of their difficulties are additional and important pieces of information. Most people evolve a model to explain their current distress. It is useful to know to what extent they are postulating threatening or progressive deterioration, undiagnosed problems, or recognition of the influence of psychological variables on pain levels. An open-ended question about the causes of their current problems will give a clue as to the extent to which they have been led to believe that they are "making it up" or that the pain is "all in the mind." With this knowledge, the therapist is better able to present the treatment to them and to know what types of anxieties need to be recognized and allayed. Catastrophic or helpless cognitions sometimes emerge at this stage. The extent to which the patient feels able to influence the pain is ascertained.

The latter part of the interview deals with the pain problem in a much more general manner, drawing on information on upbringing, family attitudes to pain, childhood illnesses and concerns over pain, psychiatric history and current problems, marital history and any relevant current difficulties. In addition, an attempt is made to assess the effects of the pain problem upon the patient's family (e.g., the reaction of the spouse or partner to pain problems, changes in spouse activities, changes in the patient's behavior when in pain, responses of family members to pain behavior or well behavior).

In considering the psychological correlates of the pain problem, it is important to evaluate the level of depression, as well as the level of anxiety or panic, and to rule out a number of other issues that might interfere with treatment: dementia (memory or intellectual deficits), intense social problems, feelings of persecution, psychotic symptomatology, obsessional illness, and fear of illness (over and above the usual somatizing tendency of chronic pain patients).

A work history is undertaken in order to evaluate the extent to which there were any difficulties or problems with respect to work prior to the pain problem; the extent to which pain has prevented or reduced the person's capacity to work; the legal implications of the disability with respect to the capacity to earn a living; and his/her current financial status. Clarify whether a return to past employment is feasible or acceptable to the patient. Sometimes the development of a chronic pain problem provokes a reexamination of career options.

A number of open-ended questions can be useful in assessing patients' motivation to change, their understanding of the psychological approach, and their expectations of the clinic. Patients with specific desires as to what they plan to do if their problems are rectified are often good candidates for this type of approach, contrasting with those patients who would behave in exactly the same manner, even if pain-free. However, this assumption has not been rigorously assessed to date and has some obvious limitations. Allow time for a discussion of the psychological treatment that is available and the suitability of the patient for such an approach.

Many pain clinics interview a spouse, friend, or relation in addition to the chronic pain patient. This information amplifies that given by the patient, providing a firsthand report of the effect of the pain problem on others. Although such information is of interest, it may prove unnecessary for the outpatient management of chronic pain, where the aim of the program is to make the patient the primary instigator of change and the discoverer of imbalances in his or her life and relationships. This manual does not include a spouse interview as a necessary component in pain management. However, it may prove to be useful with other types of patients (those in litigation, inpatients). From the clinician's point of view, the danger in putting emphasis on the corroboration of reports by spouse or partner is the tendency to disvalue the problem as it is posed by the patient, seeing it instead through the eyes of a relative or friend.

Current methods emphasize the validity of the pain problem as perceived and described by the patient, and they help the patient to find more precisely how it can be contained and brought under control. More research is necessary in order to decide on the importance of familial involvement in improving the pain management technique. To date, excellent results have been produced even without the active involvement of the spouse or partner.

QUESTIONNAIRES

The second set of information comes directly from the patients themselves, in the form of questionnaires which are sent to them prior to their first visit to the clinic. It allows them to fill in a number of inventories concerning their pain problems, and to complete daily pain diaries.

The questionnaires should cover pain experience, pain behavior, pain cognitions, anxiety, depression, and the overall impact of the pain problem.

When sending this material to patients, it is important that they have a description of the service and the implications of the questionnaires. This will allow them to be as frank as possible about the repercussions and consequences of their pain problems and to systematically monitor the course of their pain over a 2-week period. A cogent and simple description of the implications of attendance at the pain clinic with respect to assessment and management is of value. In addition, informing patients at this stage about the criteria for inclusion in the program (e.g., excluding litigation cases that have yet to be brought to the attention of the GP) makes it possible for patients to decline and thus avoids the waste of effort and time.

Many questionnaires have been used in pain management work, and the exact selection will depend to some extent on the orientation of the program and the specific focus of treatment. In this case, with a cognitive-behavioral approach designed to modify avoidance behavior, cognitions and emotional reactions to pain, the selected instruments are described below. (For further details, see Appendix VI.)

Pain Experience

This can be assessed in several ways. The McGill Pain Questionnaire (Melzack, 1975; Melzack, 1983) is a well-established instrument that is widely used in clinical and research work. It is an adjective list that allows a differentiation of sensory and affective, as well as evaluative, components of the pain experience. Despite some psychometric problems, it is an indispensable instrument for the assessment of pain. It is quickly administered and useful for obtaining an indication of the relative intensity of different aspects of the pain experience.

The limitations of questionnaires become particularly evident as the person's problem moves from a continuous to an episodic pattern, or for people who are enduring episodic problems. Sufferers tend to complete the questionnaire by drawing on their *memories* of difficult episodes, or from remembered episodes, even though their frequency may be greatly reduced by treatment. However, as initial assessment devices they are valuable for providing the adjectival descriptors that are most appropriate for the person, as well as giving an indication of the pain intensity and the degree of distress produced by the pain.

The diary method of assessing pain experience is essential. It was originally devised by Budzynski, Stoyva, and Adler (1973) and has been modified to provide average levels of distress suffered by patients during their waking hours. They are asked to monitor for 2 weeks prior to the behavioral assessment. It is assumed that the 2 weeks are characteristic of their problem, but patients should be questioned about this on receipt of the booklets. An additional 2 weeks of monitoring may be necessary if the 2-week period was exceptional (for example, if the person had flu during this period). These booklets provide daily records of the intensity of pain on a 0–5 scale through each hour of the day; they allow a daily and weekly profile to be derived and its relationship to medication intake to be evaluated. Figure 6.2 is an example of one page of a 7-page booklet, which can be made to fit into a pocket or handbag of a patient.

Some patients prefer to define their own intervals, but the majority seem content with this scale based on the interruption of daily activity (i.e., by pain). They are asked to fill it in as often as possible in the day, so that they are not depending on memory. If this proves a problem, they are asked to do it at meal times. They circle the hour when they wake and when they go to sleep, so that the estimate of pain can be derived through their waking hours. This also allows the therapist to see the extent of nighttime awakening and the levels of pain recorded at these times. The top line is used for indications of medication use. It allows the psychologist to evaluate the effect of medication, the rate of use, and its relationship to pain levels.

The pain diaries are scored in the following manner:

- Daily waking pain averages (*intensity*): the sum of rated intensities divided by waking hours (see Figure 6.2). These can be averaged each day and then accumulated to give a weekly average pain level.
- Average daily pain *duration* over one week can be obtained by counting the number of hours per day and dividing by 7.

- *Frequency* count over the period of time being analyzed can be achieved by counting the number of days in which pain episodes occur, or the number of episodes per week.
- The *average number of medications* (prescribed or nonprescribed) used per day can be calculated and averaged over the time evaluated (e.g., 2 weeks). The timing of medication use and its dependence on pain level will be made clear.
- Amount of *sleep disturbance* per week.
- Rough estimates of *variability* (peaks and troughs). These can be made more precise for research purposes by using a statistical measure of variability (standard deviation or variance).

The diary is a more accurate evaluation of the pain level suffered by a person than his or her average as estimated in the structured interview. It is calibrated hourly on his or her own scale but is anchored to a top point described as "incapacitating." Often the oral report is influenced by patients' desire to gain treatment or their memory of the worst episodes in the past few days. When depressed, the negative biasing in oral judgment may be even more exaggerated.

The program described in this manual is not likely to be effective with people who show considerable phasic variation in the pain levels (peaks and troughs). The variability allows patients to utilize strategies at key times when they need additional help to cope with peaks (episode control). Troughs are useful times to practice new skills or work on preventive strategies.

Cognitive Tests

The introduction of cognitive concepts into pain management programs created a need for new measuring instruments. The need is now being met, and several forms of cognitive assessment are under development (e.g., Edwards, Pearce, Turner-Stokes, & Jones, 1992). At present there is no single test that can be selected as the most suitable, but as norms are accumulated and tests of reliability and validity are completed, it will be possible to recommend the best measures for clinical and for research purposes.

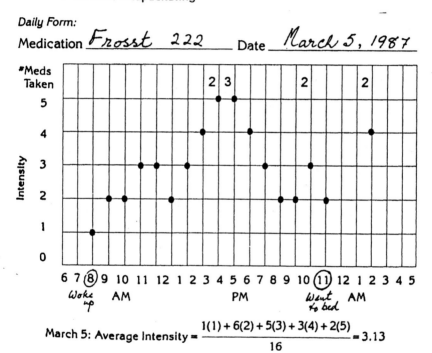

Name: _Celia Gaites_

Scale: 0 no pain
1 very low level; aware of it only at times
2 pain level can be ignored at times
3 painful, but can continue work
4 severe, makes concentration difficult
5 intense, incapacitating

Daily Form:

Medication _Frosst 222_   Date _March 5, 1987_

March 5: Average Intensity $= \dfrac{1(1) + 6(2) + 5(3) + 3(4) + 2(5)}{16} = 3.13$

FIGURE 6.2 Example of one day of a pain diary.

The development work completed so far has unearthed two main groups of cognitions. The first set pertains to beliefs about the possibilities and value of using positive coping tactics and the second set consists of negative cognitions of helplessness or an inclination to catastrophize about the significance of the pain and its enduring interference on one's life.

The negative cognitions resemble those discovered years ago in the study of depression. Catastrophizing and a sense of helplessness feature prominently in virtually all analyses of depression, posing another reminder of the common association between chronic pain and depression.

It has been found necessary to assess specific, *personal* cognitions about pain, and also *general* cognitions regarding the nature of pain and its relation to health. These general and specific cognitions are correlated but do not measure quite the same ideas, and information about both is necessary in carrying out CBT. They are necessary for helping the patients to understand, and improve, their grasp of pain phenomena, and because of the important functional connections between cognitions and behavior. The presence of deeply held negative cognitions tends to prevent or undermine the behavioral changes that are required for progress. And therapeutic progress, in turn, is best gauged by measures of cognitions, behavior, and reports of pain intensity and duration.

Psychometric scales have been developed for the measurement of pain-related cognitions, positive and negative, but for the most part they are ad hoc scales constructed for particular studies. An "all-purpose" set of cognitive measures of pain, comparable in scope and use to the McGill Pain Questionnaire, has yet to be established and adopted.

The range of published cognitive scales is indicated by this brief review of recent studies, chosen to illustrate the points made earlier about the main cognitive factors, the need for personal and general items, the relation to depressive cognitions, and so forth. Flor, Behle, and Birbaumer (1993) constructed two related self-report scales for measuring pain-related cognitions in patients with chronic pain. The first scale measures the person's cognitions about his or her specific pains and their fluctuations, and the second measures attitudes toward pain *in general*. The reliability and validity of the scales, tested on samples of 279 patients with various types of chronic pain and 38 controls, are reassuringly high, and the authors extracted four stable factors. Two factors pertaining to negative cognitions, helplessness and catastrophizing, come up in one form or another in other psychometric studies and are emerging as the potentially important cognitive "clusters." In the Flor et al. (1993) scales, key items in the *helplessness* factor included: "I cannot influence the pain"; "I am powerless, only medicine and doctors can help"; "I am worried about the future."

Key items in the *catastrophizing* factor include: "I cannot stand pain, pain drives me crazy"; "pain will never stop"; "I am a hopeless case." The catastrophizing subscale alone accounted for 33% of the variance on pain severity, and rose to 35.4% with the addition of the helplessness subscale. Scores on these scales of negative cognitions declined after successful therapy. The authors carefully analyzed the relations between the negative cognitions and depression, sometimes reported to be inextricably interwoven, and found that although depression and cognitions were positively correlated, the relation of the main factor (catastrophizing) to pain severity "is not principally explained by the mediating effect of depression" (Flor et al., 1993, p. 71).

In addition to the two factors of negative cognitions, they extracted two positive factors: resourcefulness and active coping, but found that neither of the positives were related importantly and solely to pain. The patients and controls obtained similar scores on the positive scales, and improvements after therapy were not associated with the positive scales. They did not increase with successful treatment, whereas the negative cognition scores decreased.

Boston, Pearce, and Richardson (1990) studied the cognitions that 90 mixed chronic pain patients reported *during* episodes of pain and obtained comparable results. Their investigation yielded four separable factors, two negative and two positive. The negative factors pertained to feelings of helplessness, and feelings of hopelessness, and both of these were independently correlated with pain intensity and pain distress (between 0.21 and 0.29). The key items on the hopelessness factor were: thoughts about not being able to tolerate the pain any longer, worrying about becoming a burden to family and friends, and not wanting to wake up in the morning. The main items of the helplessness factor were: pessimism about the effects of further treatment, concern about the lack of care and concern felt about others. The main conclusion from the study was that there is an association between the report of negative cognitions and both the intensity and affective dimensions of pain, albeit not a very strong association.

Other confirmation of the centrality of feelings of helplessness, and the importance of a sense of controllability of the pain, comes from a study of 62 patients with chronic low back pain (Keefe, Crisson, Urban, & Williams, 1990). A feeling of helplessness accounted for 50% of the variance in psychological stress. This finding is consistent with a number of other studies in which patients who feel that they have little or no control over their chronic pain tend to be among the most depressed and distressed patients. In a similar vein to Keefe et al. (1990) and using comparable methods of assessment, Spinhoven and Linssen (1991) found that reductions in pain and improvements in behavior and emotional adjustment were significantly correlated with changes in coping strategies and cognitions at the end of a 10-week treatment program. The authors attached particular importance to the patients' belief that they were able to exert some control over the pain.

In an investigation of the relation between pain and depression, Lefebvre (1981) produced evidence of general cognitive distortions among a group of patients with low back pain, with or without accompanying depression. Although he found clear evidence of cognitive errors among these patients (such as catastrophizing, overgeneralizing), a comparison group of people who had depression *without* accompanying pain showed the same degree of cognitive distortions. The study also produced some additional evidence of an association between chronic pain and depression, but suggested that the cognitive distortions were more likely to be a function of the depression as such, rather than the pain. A similar relation between depression and memory for pain was obtained by Eich, Rachman, and Lopatka (1990).

Pain Behavior

With the introduction of behavior therapy into the management of chronic pain, attention turned to pain-related behavior (Philips, 1987a), and a list of common forms of such behavior is reproduced in Appendix VI. Most scales of pain behavior take the form of self-reports, but clinical ratings also play a part (e.g., Fordyce, 1974).

Vlaeyen and Pernots (1990) concentrated on the *social* aspects of pain behavior and constructed a global rating scale that was used by nurses on an in-patient unit. The staff rated the behavior of 152 in-patients, and factor analysis of these ratings resulted in six factors, the most important of which were distorted mobility, "verbal complaints," and "nonverbal complaints." There were lesser factors pertaining to anxiety and depression. The results are compatible with the wider classifications used by

Turk, Wack, and Kearns (1985) who were able to classify pain behavior, social and nonsocial, into three dimensions: withdrawal, high/low arousal, and visible/audible stimulation.

The connection between the patient's cognitions and behavior is demonstrated by the fact that poor behavioral persistence on various tasks is associated with the patient having a negative view of his or her abilities, and an expectation of increased pain if they perform the physical exercises. Their psychological impairments and physical disabilities are partly the result of negative cognitions and pessimistic predictions. (See Turk & Rudy, 1992.)

The connection between beliefs and behavior is well illustrated in an interesting investigation of *beliefs* that patients have about their experiences. Williams and Thorn (1989) found evidence for two prominent pain beliefs: that pain is enduring, and that pain is mysterious. Patients who strongly endorsed these beliefs were less likely to use psychological coping strategies and inclined to catastrophize about their pain problem. By contrast, those patients who did not express strong agreement with these beliefs were more likely to use psychological coping techniques and showed less of a tendency to catastrophize. These findings emphasize the importance of the educational elements of the pain management program in overcoming common beliefs, such as these, which can impede behavioral and general progress if left unexamined.

To conclude, there is good reason to include cognitive assessments in preparing and evaluating CBT. There appear to be two separable clusters of cognitions, positive and negative, with the latter more closely related to treatment response. The negative cognitions follow the themes of helplessness and catastrophizing, and bear a resemblance to depressive cognitions. The connections between cognitions, especially the negative ones, and behavior, are functional and will influence response to treatment.

As a guide to recent work on measurement, a list of selected references, plus a list of common cognitions, is included in Appendix VI.

Measures of More Pervasive Consequences

In addition to these instruments, which are intended to assess the pain problem per se, a number of other instruments are useful. The Beck

Depression Inventory (Beck, Ward, Mendelson, Mock, & Erbaugh, 1961) is recommended as a useful measure of depression, and is now widely used in pain management research (Beck, Steer, & Garbin, 1988). Scores between 10–15 indicate mild depression; between 16–30 moderate depression; and scores above 30 indicate severe depression.

Anxiety levels can be quickly assessed using the State Trait Anxiety Inventory (Spielberger, 1983) and amplified with the Fear Survey Schedule (Tomlin et al., 1984) if specific anxieties are present. Because of the increasing invasion of pain into every aspect of a person's life, the Sickness Impact Profile (Bergner, Bobbitt, Carter, & Gilson, 1981) may be of use in providing a survey for the clinician of the disruptive effects of pain, across a number of domains. The patient can fill it out quickly, and it can be useful for the clinician both in focusing discussion in the interview and in providing an overall measure of disruption.

These inventories have been selected to amplify the description of a specific pain problem (experience and behavior, behavior and cognitions) as well as to compare the level of depression and anxiety in pain and in pain-free populations. No personality measures are necessary. No particular personality types have been shown to be specifically vulnerable to chronic pain problems or particularly responsive to psychological treatments. Personality inventories are designed to evaluate enduring personality characteristics, rather than the specific effects of the current pain problem upon which the treatment is focused. For these reasons no particular benefit is gained by including a personality assessment in selecting patients for this type of treatment.

INTEGRATION OF ASSESSMENT INFORMATION

The psychologist coordinating the pain service must make specific decisions about the people assessed and their suitability for psychological treatment. The integration of the material collected is illustrated in Figure 6.1 (p. 59). It can be seen that the first level of nonacceptance occurs with the referral to the clinic, where a referring physician may indicate facts about patients that would eliminate them from consideration (''Exclusionary Criteria,'' mentioned previously). If, however, patients appear to be suitable candidates, they are then interviewed, and results of the structured interview are integrated with those from the pain diary and questionnaires.

The daily diary rating of pain, over a 2-week period, is a more reliable estimate of the typical levels of pain, use of analgesics, sleep patterns, and the fluctuations of pain than is the information recalled by the patient at the interview. Inconsistencies between these two estimates can be dealt with on the spot during the interview, and they often produce interesting amplifications of the patient's problem. The behavioral questionnaire can save interview time, as it surveys the relevant pain behavior. Inconsistencies may be found between the results on this questionnaire and self-report in sessions, particularly where compensation or litigation is involved. These inconsistencies are, once again, interesting ones to be taken up in the session by the psychologist. The responses on the questionnaires may be a measure of a patient's desire to demonstrate a problem, rather than a direct reflection of his or her behavioral avoidance and incapacity. Using the questionnaires and the structured interview, the psychologist can then make a decision with respect to the positive criteria listed previously.

However, the final decision, with respect to suitability for treatment, cannot be made by the psychologist alone. The physician, pharmacist, or physical therapist may find reason for faulting the selection. The patient may have been inadequately evaluated, may have too great a drug dependence to be managed on an outpatient basis, or may need a more (or less) intensive physical therapy program. These types of reasons may make the program impractical or impossible for the patient, despite his or her acceptability from a psychological point of view. It can be seen from Figure 6.1 that the decision concerning suitability for treatment is sequential. Integration of the different sources of information is necessary in order to arrive at the final decision with respect to suitability for treatment.

TREATMENT FORMAT

The majority of chronic pain patients can be treated as well, if not better, in a group than treated individually. Group treatment allows the training to focus on pain management and reduces the tendency of many people to persist in focusing on their own somatic complaints. In fact, the group acts as an important social inhibitor of repeated self-examination and complaint. Pain patients are not interested in the complaints of others, and their lack of interest is inhibitory. Many chronic pain patients who are actively avoiding involvement in life and have reduced their level of exercise and activity, find themselves lonely and isolated. This contributes to their problems. Bringing them into a group immediately counteracts this, and enables them to make normal social contact with people who have an understanding of their difficulty. Working alongside other people with comparable problems (chronic pain) focuses attention on the similarities of their psychological responses to pain despite the differences in etiology, history chronicity, sensation, and so forth.

In a group with other sufferers, the patient begins to witness the importance of active attempts to evolve appropriate strategies. Individual differences in the effects of strategies can be drawn out by the therapist over the nine weeks. This process encourages each participant to experiment between sessions and to define which strategies are useful for him or her.

Group pressure can be a positive motivating force in increasing adherence to such regimes as increased exercise and reduced medication. In addition, the pressure can be a positive impetus to test and evaluate the strategies discussed. Homework is discussed at the beginning of each session, allowing this group pressure to be wielded. It becomes an increasing embarrassment for persons to report that they have not completed their homework tasks, and the praise of the group acts as a potent motivational force in encouraging group members to undertake assignments. Because all members of the group are not at the same stage of pain management, the ones further ahead in the utilization of strategies act as models for those who are trailing behind or are having difficulty with learning a particular strategy. In addition, members of the group may comment on particular difficulties they have in the utilization of some strategy and how to overcome them or how to exploit the value of the strategy. Information from group members has a powerful impact upon other members of the group, and modeling occurs in these sessions. However, there are a number of important provisos that need to be made to this positive outlook on the cost-effective method of group treatment of chronic pain problems. The workings of the group can be disrupted by patients whose problems are of too great a magnitude to allow them to concentrate on pain management techniques (e.g., major marital discord, depression). In selection, it is important to exclude people whose capacity to join constructively into the treatment approach is in doubt. Excessively anxious or unassertive people may find the group work distressing, and sometimes it is necessary for them to undergo some type of social skills training *prior* to working in a group. Individual treatment for pain may be more appropriate for them, unless they can first resolve their social difficulties.

Patients with severe physical handicaps as well as pain may find the physical demands of the program too great and should be excluded (e.g., those incapable of walking, swimming, or bicycling, or those unable to hear or see). Extremely aggressive, hostile, and destructive people are not recommended for group therapy. They may require a good deal of therapist attention in order to prevent them from undermining the work of the group, and are best dealt with on their own rather than in a group.

The group discussions facilitate exploration of negative cognitions and their evaluation by a group of fellow sufferers. This is an unusually influential source of relevant information and informed opinions.

PREPARATION FOR TREATMENT

The first interview can be critical. Many patients come to psychological treatment programs unwillingly—skeptical, frustrated, and even angry, feeling that they have been fobbed off as complainers, fakers, or even worse, as mentally disturbed. Many feel, and with justification, that health care services, sometimes including the referring agent, fail to believe in the authenticity of their pain. The referral is interpreted as a sign that their pain is erroneously regarded as imaginary or even faked. And imaginary pains, or exaggerated or faked pains, lie in the province of psychology, not infrequently confused with psychiatry, in which case the referral can be interpreted as indicating that the patient may be mentally ill.

Many patients arrive with the strong belief that their pain has a physical basis, in the form of an injury, disease or dysfunction, and that relief depends on the detection of *the cause* of the pain. The persistence of the pain is interpreted as a failure of diagnosis, as a failure to find the hidden cause of the pain. Of course, this network of powerful, unexamined beliefs, rests on the outdated specificity theory of pain with its assumption of a direct, simple relation between injury and pain. Hence, the failure of health care services to detect and diagnose the hidden cause of the pain is interpreted as evidence of incompetence, or worse, an ominous sign of a rare and potentially serious disease.

It will be appreciated that in these circumstances, many patients approach their first meeting with a psychologist without enthusiasm. Given that they regard the referral as wrong, annoyance, skepticism, and resentment are understandable. So is their disinclination to listen to a radically different, *psychological* view of pain, based as they believe, on a lack of appreciation of their problem. The idea that pain is extremely complex and that the relation between injury and pain is highly variable, seems at first to be irrelevant to their needs.

Hence, it is best to encourage patients to describe their medical experiences in their own words, and to express their beliefs about the nature of their problem and the nature of pain itself. The psychologist then introduces the new information, including teaching material, and elicits from the patient examples of how emotional change affects their pain. The therapist then introduces the pretreatment educational video.

Video Modeling

The powerful effects of psychological modeling are well established, and these effects are facilitated by the use of coping models who are similar to the observer. In cases of chronic pain, observing a video in which earlier patients with comparable pain problems, and similar medical experiences, describe and discuss their initial explanations and beliefs about pain, provides a valuable educational experience. The video, prepared on site, to ensure similarity to future patients, shows the changing beliefs and understanding of the pain patients as they progress through the program. The video should also include at least one example of unsuccessful treatment.

The use of earlier, comparable patients as the models for new patients is an expeditious and convincing means of facilitating a deeper understanding of pain in general, and one's own pain in particular. It can promote such understanding equally well or more quickly than purely didactic sessions with a therapist can do on their own. If the video is shown to a newly formed group of patients, it can provoke a valuable exchange of experiences and beliefs about pain, followed by a discussion of modern views about pain.

Following the structured interview and completion of the questionnaires, the patient's attention is focused on selected aspects of the problem (e.g., lack of active coping strategies, behavioral limitations). As a consequence, it is an easy step to initiate a discussion of how coping strategies can be learned and active control over the pain problem increased. The goal becomes one of regaining a more normal life with diminishing interference from the pain.

It should not be assumed that the physicians have had time to explain the program to the patients. Therefore the psychologist should provide a concise and factual description of the program to the patient, giving the content and emphasis, as well as the rough percentage of patients who have improved using these techniques. Approximately 70% to 80% of patients treated are clinically improved, with a smaller percentage pain-free or virtually pain-free. Because of the different types of problems, different amounts of residual damage, inherited weaknesses, and so forth, the amount of improvement will vary between patients. However, the factual material allows the patient to begin to form appropriate expectations about what he or she may be able to achieve.

In addition, prepare the patient so that he or she understands the time course of treatment and its nature (i.e., skill training). Emphasize the fact that patients are going to be learning techniques that need to be practiced. The more practiced, the better able they will be to use the strategy when dealing with pain. The treatment weeks initiate a process that the therapist expects will increment gradually over the months following treatment. Each session is described to the patient as adding a piece of a jigsaw, which, when they have completed the full treatment program, will form a picture. With this "picture," they will have a greater understanding of their pain problem and how to manage it. In the weeks following treatment the patients will be using the techniques and gradually improving their skills. The importance of regular attendance at sessions should be emphasized, and here the image of a jigsaw puzzle may be useful. Patients who miss a place in the jigsaw may not see the image in the total picture.

It is useful to show prospective group members a video of patients during their reassessment interview and a follow-up 6 months or even a year later. It gives them valuable information about the nature of pain and how the program operates. Being able to listen to other patients summarizing their experiences in the pain management sessions can be an important and powerful therapeutic tool. A library of such cases is a valuable asset, allowing the effects of modeling to be mobilized in strengthening the motivation for a self-management approach. As yet, a full investigation of the role of modeling per se in the management of chronic pain has not been undertaken, but it is likely that observational learning will be as strong in this area as has been manifest in other clinical settings.

It is important for the therapist to make clear the demands that will be made on the patient. Full attendance and intensive work *between* sessions is crucial to the effectiveness of the treatment techniques. In addition, required attendance at a posttreatment reassessment and follow-up must be made clear. Apart from delineating the changes made by the patient, these follow-ups can act as important incentives and booster sessions by giving the patient a perspective that includes follow-up visits and reinforces the idea of progressive changes and the gradual evolution of skills.

All patients are asked to formulate goals for themselves in negotiation with the therapist. These are made for short periods of time. The first goals are set at the onset of treatment and span the nine weeks of treatment. The second set is made at the posttreatment assessment and covers the two months until follow-up. Finally, new goal sheets are prepared by the patients at follow-up to take them up to one year posttreatment. Emphasis is placed on the specific nature of these goals and on the necessity for being realistic. In fact, the filling in of a goal sheet becomes the first stage in therapeutic management; it will be discussed in Chapter 7. It is mentioned here because of the role of goal sheets can play in preparing the patient to undertake an active self-management approach to the pain problem.

SUGGESTED READINGS

Beck, A. T., Ward, C. H., Mendelson, M., Mock, J., & Erbaugh, J. (1961). An inventory for measuring depression. *Archives of General Psychiatry, 4,* 53–63.

Beck, A., Steer, R., & Garbin, M. (1988). Psychometric properties of the Beck Depression Inventory. *Clinical Psychology Review, 8,* 77–100.

Bergner, M., Bobbitt, R. A., Carter, W. B., & Gilson, B. S. (1981). The sickness impact profile: Development and final revision of a health status measure. *Medical Care, 19,* 787–805.

Block, A. (1980). Behavioral treatment of chronic pain: Variables affecting treatment efficacy. *Pain, 8,* 367–375.

Budzynski, T. H., Stoyva, J. M., & Adler, C. (1973). EMG biofeedback and tension headache. *Psychosomatic Medicine, 35,* 484–496.

Derebury, J., & Tullis, W. H. (1983). Delayed recovery in patients with work compensation injuries. *Journal of Occupational Medicine, 125*(11), 829–835.

Dworkin, R. H., Handlin, D. S., Richlin, D. M., Brand, L., & Vannucci, C. (1985). Unravelling the effects of compensation, litigation, and employment on treatment response in chronic pain. *Pain, 23,* 49–59.

Follick, M. J., Zitter, R. E., & Ahern, D. K. (1983). Failures in operant treatment of chronic pain. In E. B. Foa & P. M. G. Emmelkamp (Eds.), *Failures in behavior therapy* (pp. 311–334). New York: Wiley.

Hammonds, W., Brenner, F., & Unikel, J. P. (1974). Compensation for work related injuries and rehabilitation of patients with chronic pain. *STH Medical Journal, 71,* 664–666.

Hunter, M. (1983). The Headache Scale: A new approach to the assessment of headache pain based on pain descriptors. *Pain, 16,* 361–373.

Melzack, R. (1975). The McGill Pain Questionnaire: Major properties and scoring methods. *Pain, 1,* 277–299.

Melzack, R. (Ed.). (1983). *Pain measurement and assessment.* NY: Raven Press.

Penzien, M. S., Holroyd, K. A., Holm, J. E., & Hursey, K. G. (1985). Psychometric characteristics of Bakal Headache Assessment Questionnaire. *Headache, 25*(1), 55–58.

Philips, H. C. (1987). Thoughts provoked by pain. *Behavior Research & Therapy, 27,* 469–474.

Philips, H. C., & Jahanshahi, M. (1986). The components of pain behavior report. *Behavior Research and Therapy, 24*(2), 117–125.

Roberts, A. H., & Reinhardt, L. (1980). Behavioral management of chronic pain: Long-term follow-up with comparison groups. *Pain, 8,* 151–162.

Spielberger, C. (1983). *Manual for the State-Trait Anxiety Inventory.* Palo Alto,
CA: Consulting Psychologists Press.

Tomlin, P., Thyer, B. A., Curtis, G. C., Nesse, R., Camero, D., & Wright,
P. (1984). Standardization of the FSS. *Journal of Behavior Therapy and
Experimental Psychiatry, 15,* 123–126.

Trief, P., & Stein, N. (1985). Pending litigation and rehabilitation outcome of
chronic back pain. *Archives of Physical Medicine and Rehabilitation,
66*(2), 95–99.

PART II
Treatment

Introduction

Each of the nine sessions is discussed in a separate chapter. As in the sessions, the chapters consist of five parts:

1. homework review
2. didactic presentation
3. introduction of tactics and practice
4. homework assignments
5. suggested readings.

In addition, solutions to some of the more common problems that arise for the therapist are included in separate subsections within each chapter.

Figure 7.1 (p. 85) lays out the full 9-week treatment program, showing the timing of the introduction of each of the tactics and their relationship to the didactic presentation. The latter focuses on factors known to affect the level of pain experienced or the development of vicious cycles that can amplify pain. The tactics are ways in which a person can gain control over his or her pain problem, in breaking vicious cycles, and in diminishing pain experience and increasing tolerance for pain.

CHAPTER 7

Orientation: Chronic Pain and the Self-Management Approach (Session #1)

INTRODUCTION AND GOAL SETTING

This first session is a crucial one. It prepares the way for all the work that will be undertaken in the subsequent eight weeks, and provides the explanation of the type of approach being taught.

Prior to introducing the program, encourage the members of the group to introduce themselves. A useful way of undertaking introductions is to ask each person to describe briefly the nature of the problem he or she is seeking help with, and the length of time they have been enduring it.

Another introduction to the self-management approach comes from asking each member of the group to establish realistic and specific goals to be achieved during the subsequent eight weeks. It is often the case that chronic pain patients find it very difficult to think of what they would like to do, their thoughts being so dominated by the one idea: How can

I stop the pain? It is important to begin to shift this focus and to start the process of constructive thinking about what they would like to achieve during the treatment period. A prolonged pain problem disrupts every area of life: work, leisure, relationships, sleep, capacity and willingness to exercise, and so forth. It is hard for sufferers to think of any activity that has not been adversely affected. The pain becomes a tyrant, ruling them and controlling their actions and plans.

The goal sheet can be explained at the onset of this first session, and the discussion is aided if the goal sheets are precirculated to participants at their final assessment sessions. They will have been able to discuss their hopes and predictions with their families and give some constructive thought to what they may be able to achieve. If it has not been possible to provide the sheets prior to this session, so begin work in the session by asking patients to complete them for the next week. The discussion can take place during the usual homework review section (see Figure 7.1) or can be shifted to the end of the tactics practice section, whichever seems more satisfactory.

An example of a goal sheet is provided in Figure 7.2. It is important to emphasize to patients that they need to find at least one goal under each of the headings and to fill in their goals without reference to pain or distress. The goals should be realistic. A goal that can be broken up into parts and then approached gradually is the best kind to encourage. With respect to exercise, for example, discourage goals such as "run a mile." This is guaranteed to make them fail. A more realistic goal may be "exercise (walking briskly) for 20 consecutive minutes per day." It is important for the goals to be specific. For example, the initial thought that the patient would like to "learn a new skill" should be redefined as to "learn tailoring by attending one evening class per week" or to "work in the garden for two hours a day."

Encourage the patients to choose at least one activity they wish to achieve in each of the areas. "Work" does not necessarily mean a paid occupation, but includes voluntary work or part-time work; and housework is, of course, considered as relevant in this category as paid work outside the house.

Leisure activities are often curtailed or reduced by chronic pain patients. Encourage them to begin thinking constructively about the gradual return to some of these activities or the development of new interests that are

	1	2	3	4	5	6	7	8	9
Homework Review	Goal Sheets	Basal Exercise levels set; Problems re breathing task resolved	Reactions to tape use, exercise, and regular drug sched; Problems? Conc. re self-monitored pain patterns	Reactions to liquid equivalent re drugs using Pain Diaries - exercise - relaxation; Conc. re self-monitored pain and individual patterning	Reactions to drug reduction, exercise increase and relax; Conclusion re stress events for each patient	Reactions to HW; Conclusions re assertiveness; Cond. re spouse/patient monitor; N.B. discrepancies Problems	Reactions to HW; Success re negotiations with spouse and assertion (reactions of family); Conc. re self-talk	Reactions to HW tasks; Conclusions re avoidance/confrontation monitoring	Reactions to HW; Conclusions re pacing problems and individual differences in strategy use
Didactic	Orientation to self-management approach and presentation of gate control framework	Role of relaxation in pain management (Negative role of muscular response)	Role of exercise/activity levels	Role of drugs (side effects, tolerance, etc.)	Role of emotional state - anxiety - anger	Role of attention focus & complaint; Indirect demonstration of needs (and complaint) - the need for assertion	Role of appraisal of pain and depression	Role of activity pacing	Review of individual differences - episodic vs preventative strategy - adapt of others to pt changes - dealing with setbacks
Strategy Introduction/Practice	Strategy 1A; Diaphragmatic breathing	Strategy 1B; Progressive relaxation (with breath control) (10 muscle group)	Strategy 2; Specific exercise and/or clarification re general exercise choice/requirement	Strategy 5; Relaxation and distracting imagery; Strategy 3; Drug reduction	Strategy 4; Delusing/reducing stress reactions	Strategy 5; Focusing tech Distraction; Strategy 6; Assertion role-play (if necessary)	Strategy 7; Cue-controlled relaxation; Strategy 8; Reappraisal and self-talk techniques	Strategy 9; Activity pacing; Strategy 7; Cue control (continued)	Strategy 1 - 9; Practise of any technique req; Emphasis on episodic tech use and short relaxation induction (6 min or less); Examination of Goal Sheets
Assignment of Homework	*Practise breath control 2 times daily; *Monitor exercise to establish onset level	*Practise relaxation with tape (2 times daily); *Exercise daily at basal level; *Take medication 3-4 times daily by the clock	*Activity increment; *Relaxation (2 x daily); *Liquid equivalent drug regime begins; *Pain diaries	*Exercise up; *Relaxation; *Drug reduction to 90%; *Monitor stressful events in Pain Diary	*Exercise up, drugs to 75%; *Relax (cue); *Delusing skill indicate success, etc. on self-talk; *Spouse & patient to monitor pain talk/actions indep; *Assertion disc. test	*Drugs to 55%; Exercise up; Relax. regular; *Disc. communication & spouse responses to compliant, with spouse; *Assertion exercise; *Cease Diaries; *Monitor self-talk	*Drugs to 35%; Exercise up; Relax. reg & short self-talk; *Increase pleasurable activities (see goal sheet); *Use reappraisal techniques; *Monitor avoidance actions	*Drugs to 15%; Exercise up; Relaxation; *Reduced avoidance/confrontation; *Cue control; *Compare strategy monitoring	*Drugs to 0%; Exercise up; Actives up; *Goal sheets for 8 week F U; *Diaries for one wk

*Sessional Homework Assigment   *Preparation Homework Assigment

FIGURE 7.1 Layout of weekly treatment program.

85

Name: *Celia Gaites*   Date: *March*

GOAL PLANNING

A. Work
   1. *Clear away dishes + help with dishwashing. (4-5x wk)*
   2. *Start voluntary work 2 days/wk*
   3. *Arrange part-time work to start in 2nd month of treatment program*

B. Pleasurable/Leisure Activities
   1. *Prepare seed trays of vegetable seeds*
   2. *Read 4 (fiction) books*
   3. *Sand + finish bookshelf*

C. Daily Exercise
   1. *Walk briskly once/day for 30 min.*
   2. *Complete flexion exercises daily (up to 10 x each)*
   3. *Return to swimming gradually (to 2 x wk for 20 min/occasion).*

D. Social Activities
   1. *Phone 2 friends/wk*
   2. *Arrange one social event with family (wk)*
   3. *Go bowling every other week*

E. Other
   1. *Get up + dress by 8:30 each day*
   2. *Reduce day rest to nil*
   3. *Reduce (or eliminate) use of my pain pills.*

FIGURE 7.2 Example of goal sheet.

86

more in keeping with their current capacity. It is important to increase enjoyable activities on a daily basis. Discourage their inclusion in the goal sheets of activities related to pain management ("going to the chiropractor"), even if this is enjoyable to them at present.

It is essential that they include an *exercise* goal that is to be achieved during the treatment period. If no physical therapist is available to advise on particular goals, a reasonable achievement would be 20 to 30 minutes of sustained brisk walking daily. If they already undertake such an activity, they can be encouraged to incorporate new activities, such as cycling or swimming.

Chronic pain patients tend to let their friendships slip and they become isolated. It is important to halt this withdrawal and to encourage a plan to begin gradually reversing this trend during the treatment period. Again, encourage specific social goals that are realistic ("Contact two friends per week, and arrange one social activity every two weeks").

The last category is untitled and can be defined separately by each person. Individual goals that they wish to achieve over this time, or goals with respect to analgesic reduction or sleep onset, can be included in this category.

The completion of a goal sheet is an interesting task for both patients and therapist. It focuses the patients' attention on important areas in which they are encouraged to make progress. It helps them to define realistic goals for themselves. These goals will be worked toward irrespective of their current pain problems. The implied message is that *certain activities can and will be undertaken despite pain.* The techniques to be taught will enable patients to move forward to achieving these goals. The more precisely defined the goals, the easier it will be for each person to evaluate his or her success during the treatment period.

Problem Solving

It is often the case that a goal sheet is initially used as a way of expressing wishes and hopes with respect to the effect of treatment, rather than as a specific description of what can be achieved, given their current difficulty. For example, a patient who is aware of the stress he is under at work might choose to "find myself a new career." Although this may be a long-term goal, and one that is achievable, the chances of his doing so during the nine weeks of treatment are extremely slim. The therapist's aim is to encourage patients to make the goals as attainable as possible, while still requiring some change.

Some patients will complete a goal sheet with multiple goals under each entry, while others will have difficulty filling in anything at all. Both these reactions are of interest to the therapist. The first may be suggestive of excessive demandingness and lack of pacing, while the latter may be suggestive of depression or poor motivation. Keeping these tendencies in mind, the therapist should give the patient a chance to fill in a second goal sheet that takes into account the importance of realistic and specific goals. For the first person, fewer goals would be a more realistic option, perhaps taking the ones with highest priority for the patient and limiting them to three. Patients who can find nothing to put on their goal sheets can be helped by the group and by the therapist in generating specific activities to include.

It is often the case that patients fail to include drug reduction as an aim and may need reminders of other problems raised in the psychological assessment that could be included under Section E (e.g., sleep disturbance). Be careful, however, to discourage patients from including goals under Section E that will not specifically be focused on in treatment (e.g., reduction of spider phobias, reduction of obsessional rituals, weight loss). When a patient raises such possibilities it is better to suggest that these will be reassessed after treatment in the tenth week but that they are not the focus of the present treatment. The goal sheet is specifically designed to aid in treatment of chronic pain. However, it sometimes happens that other problems are improved by the increasing self-efficacy and mastery that a patient feels, and on occasion these problems diminish as an indirect consequence of treatment.

The daily exercise goal can be made precise for the patient in terms of the physical therapist's predictions of his or her physical capacity and estimates of the appropriate goal (if available). This aids the therapist in helping the patient find a realistic goal. When the patient is unwilling to shift his or her own goal and that goal is discrepant from the physical therapist's, a good approach is to have him or her write in the physical therapist's goal in a different colored ink. At the end of treatment, the patient can judge how realistic his or her hopes were and how closely they approximated the physical therapist's expectations.

It is wise to obtain a copy of the person's goal sheet, returning the original to the patient to be posted at home as a reminder to be referred to periodically during treatment.

ORIENTATION

Chronic Pain and the Inadequacy of the Acute Pain Model

The didactic presentation in this first session is of great importance. It provides the foundation for all other sessions, giving the patient a model or framework (i.e., a simplified Gate Control Model) into which he or she can fit the information received.

The details that the therapist provides about the Gate Control Model and the inadequacy of the acute approach to chronic pain, based on the specificity theory, are explained in a simple but noncondescending manner. The patients should become minor experts on the subject of chronic pain. Even the most complex subjects can be explained in simple and understandable ways (see Appendix III).

The inadequacy of the acute model for explaining chronic pain can be illustrated by using everyday examples from their own experiences. These examples are powerful in making more complex models understandable. A discussion of the failure of an athlete to notice an injury during a football game or the influence of an entirely mental intervention (hypnosis) on pain levels can help to point out the inadequacy of the acute pain model and the importance of considering a more complex explanation. The members of the group are encouraged to contribute examples of occasions when their experience was not consistent with the extent, site, and timing of physical injury, if any. They are also asked to recall episodes of pain that were not preceded or caused by injury or illness.

Physical, Emotional, and Cognitive Influences

The concept of a pain "gate" is acceptable to patients especially when theoretical discussion is kept to a minimum and practical examples are generated by the therapist or the group to illustrate the inadequacy of the acute model of pain.

Encourage the patients to discuss the influences on the gate. Begin by encouraging them to classify the negative influences on the gate, for example, those factors that make pain worse or "open the gate." These influences can be classified as: (1) physical factors, (2) emotional factors, and (3) cognitive or thinking factors.

The physical factors are the ones that most patients have given most thought to. It is useful to include the idea of residual scarring, as well as the extent of original injury (and degenerative changes). Pain can be produced when scar tissue is stretched, especially when nerve fibers have become enmeshed in the scar tissue, a fact that is not known to most pain patients. It is a comfort for them to begin to consider the possibility that the pain (for example, in the spine) might be a consequence of movements of this scar tissue, rather than a reopening of a previous wound or a worsening of their condition. In addition, a discussion of other physical factors that contribute to pain and that are nonspecific and nonprogressive in nature is useful (i.e., postural asymmetries, minor spinal stenosis, inherited instabilities in cerebral arteries, overuse of certain muscle groups). The legitimacy of a physical ingredient in the multivariate causation of pain can be pointed out without having any implications for further physical intervention. This can be emphasized by drawing upon, and discussing, such physical correlates as ischemic conditions, fibromyocitis, inflammations, and other soft tissue changes. None of these physical changes will show up on x-rays, but they may contribute to the person's experience of pain.

Finally, reflexive muscle tensing, so useful in recovering from acute injury, can become a chronic condition as pain persists posthealing. These muscular responses may contribute to the physical factors augmenting pain intensity. Virtually all chronic pain patients are aware of their guarding and anticipatory tension, especially in those parts of the body near the locus of their pain problem. It is difficult for them to relax these areas, and many describe a sense of impotence with respect to controlling the muscular responses they are experiencing. The inability of the brain to differentiate muscular guarding from muscular damage as a consequence of injury should be pointed out to patients, again giving them a model for reappraising their experiences.

By discussing physical factors first, therapists will find patients much more receptive to considering a second group of factors that can make pain worse (or "open the gate")—emotional factors. Most patients are aware of the exacerbating role that anxiety, tension, anger, and depression can play in their pain experience. These can be highlighted in the discussion by encouraging patients to describe incidents illustrating these connections. The therapist has the advantage of having completed a detailed structured interview with each of the patients in which the emotional influences were clarified. Emphasize the normality of these emotional responses to continuing pain and the likelihood that anybody would feel these emotions when their doctors are unable to help them with persisting and incapacitating pain.

Finally, introduce the role of the third set of factors in influencing the position of the gate—cognitive, or "thinking" factors. Pain tolerance is influenced by the focus of attention upon pain, distraction, boredom, and lack of stimulation as well as the attitudes or beliefs a person has about his or her pain problem. In addition, a feeling of lack of control has been shown to have a marked effect on pain tolerance. The less control a person feels over an aversive experience, the more troublesome and painful the experience. The influence of these cognitive factors is best explained by giving instances. For example, patients can be asked to compare the intensity of chest pain that occurs after supper if they believe it to be due to indigestion with the same experience if they believe the pain to be a precursor to a heart attack. Boredom felt when lying in bed in the darkness can increase the pain experienced, as the person's attention focuses on sensations. Attending to a pain, and internal focusing of attention, amplifies the pain experience.

It is necessary to spend some time on these three influences to illustrate how they can modulate pain experience in an adverse way. With this point clearly established, a fruitful discussion can be begun on the way in which these three factors can be *reversed* to reduce pain experience. Using the terminology of the Gate Control Model, the patients are seeking to find those factors that will help them to "close their gate." In this case, the physical factors are perhaps the least important of the three, with the exception of training in muscular relaxation. Other physical factors will have been explored repeatedly by physicians trying to help patients manage their pain problems prior to their coming for psychological management. Drugs will have been tried, and many patients will have experienced diminishing therapeutic effects, with increasing side-effects. Surgeries can only be undertaken on a small percentage of back pain problems, and having discussed the issue of scar tissue, many may feel much less keen on pressing for repeated surgeries. Counterstimulation is a transitory physical intervention, although its nature and effects are worth clarifying.

Thus, in summary, the positive physical factors that can be manipulated by patients in order to increase their pain tolerance are limited. However, the one available to them is extremely powerful, namely, muscular control. This tactic is taught throughout the treatment program, being introduced in Session #2.

The feasibility of utilizing emotional factors to limit, reduce, or ameliorate pain experience can then be discussed. The importance of learning how to produce a mental calm and defuse anxiety, feelings of anger and frustration can be emphasized. The important point being made is that the control of emotions can influence pain tolerance.

Finally, there are many ways in which cognitive factors can be modulated in order to affect the position of the gate and increase pain tolerance. A number of tactics will be taught during the treatment program that can be briefly mentioned at this stage (e.g., distraction, use of concentration techniques, external focusing of attention). These cognitive methods aid the patient in controlling pain levels.

The effect of the discussion of influential factors is to emphasize that chronic pain is not merely a function of physical changes or tissue damage. A number of other factors influence how much, and how often, a person feels pain.

Patients are advised that progress on all three components of the pain (cognitive, behavioral and physiological) generally is uneven at first. The three components tend to change at different rates (desynchronously—Rachman & Hodgson, 1974; Wuitchik, Bakal, & Lipshitz, 1990).

Vicious Cycles

When pain persists for long periods of time, a number of vicious cycles will develop, which paradoxically lead to increasing pain and reduced tolerance. The most common reactions to continuing pain are increasing muscle tension, guarding and disuse, anxiety, anger, depression, preoccupation, or focusing on the pain problem. From the previous discussion, it is clear that all of these reactions, although natural when pain persists, exacerbate the problem. When caught in these cycles (see Figure 7.3), often without realizing it, chronic pain patients feel increasingly impotent as to how they can break out of them. Patients often nod emphatically at this time and feel strongly that Figure 7.3 shows exactly the position they are currently in, or have been in periodically over the years.

The process of treatment can now be presented as a structured attempt to teach participants *how* to break the vicious cycles that have developed. People can learn tactics that help them to "close the gate" and reduce the sensations, or increase their pain tolerance. These tactics are under the sufferer's own control and will gain strength with repeated practice.

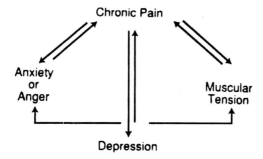

FIGURE 7.3   Vicious cycles.

Group Treatment Method

Make clear the specific requirements of the treatment program for each person (1 1/2-hour sessions weekly, homework assignments, gradual reduction of analgesics, and an increase in fitness). In addition, make clear to the patients the expectations they can develop with respect to what can be achieved during the 9-week period. Discourage them from seeking miracles or expecting sudden improvements. Remind them of the percentage of patients who improve using this method. Explain that each person's improvement depends on a great number of factors, including the extent of residual injury, if any. The best and most durable changes take place gradually and occur because participants practice coping skills and move toward an approach to their problem that is directed and controlled by themselves. Their aim should be to progress as far as they can within the period of time that they are being treated, establishing a habit of dealing with pain in a way that will become increasingly potent as they continue practicing the strategies. The analogy of learning to ride a bicycle can be useful. No one expects to ride perfectly on the first occasion, but after many practice sessions they find they have developed the skill to ride under difficult conditions (wet roads, at night, etc.). The importance of their deciding which tactic suits their particular problem is important. As yet, it is not possible to match particular tactics with particular patients.

Because of this, patients have to become active investigators of the tactics in order to discover which ones best suit them. Individual differences should be stressed. Suggest the idea of the therapist as provider of a ''smorgasbord'' of possible tactics, from which the members of the group select the most effective for their own use.

Finish by pointing out that group treatment is possible because of the similarities in the reaction of chronic pain patients to their problems despite the differences in pain locus and pain history. Chronic pain sufferers are similar in their mood changes, muscular reactions, tendency to social withdrawal or overcommitment, overactivity, or complete withdrawal from exercise and involvement. They are also similar in their reaction to other people. They may detect sympathy, anger, or dismissal in friends and relations and respond with an increasing focus on their own problems. This focusing will further ''open'' their gate. Because of these similarities, their problems can be dealt with as a group. In addition, they will benefit from the encouragement that other people suffering from pain problems can give them, as well as benefiting from the discoveries made by others about the utility of the tactics taught.

End your presentation by encouraging the discussion of many of the issues that seem unclear. Provide some written material for the patients to take home, so that they can think out the issues in more detail and discuss them with their families (see Appendix III).

Problem Solving

Individual patients may inquire into the role of diet when discussing physical factors that exacerbate pain. This is of particular interest to headache sufferers, especially if they have been given the diagnosis of migraine. Approximately 10% of the migraine population have been found to have some food allergies. It is a very small group, but nonetheless a subject of consequence to pain sufferers who would like to be able to find a simpler way of reducing migraine frequency. There is no reason why exclusionary diets may not be tried by patients, and it is a good idea to let them know, if they inquire, of the kinds of substances that have been found to be associated with migraine episodes for a *small* proportion of cases: cheese, chocolate, citrus fruit, red wine, and so forth (see Appendix VII). For the majority of cases, these dietary factors will not make any difference, but a small percentage are sensitive. It should be emphasized to them, however, that diet is just one of a number of influences on the frequency of headache. Far from being triggers for the majority of people, certain foods are contributing factors, and they may be much larger contributors under certain conditions (stage in the menstrual cycle, stage in life, premenopausal, already under stress). It is because of the complexity of these interactions that it is can be difficult to positively substantiate food allergies. However, there is nothing to be lost in patients' experimenting with dietary influences. This active attempt to classify the factors that influence their pain and to regulate them is consistent with the approach being taught. In order not to disrupt sessions, these kinds of specific factors can be described in supplementary material.

Give readings to those interested in exploring these ideas further. If many of the group suffer headaches, time can be taken during Session #4 to cover some of these issues more fully.

Orientation (Session #1)

DEEP DIAPHRAGMATIC BREATHING (TACTIC #lA)

In this first session, immediately begin teaching a specific tactic that will be utilized in conjunction with muscular relaxation training, to be introduced in the next session. The training in deep diaphragmatic breathing becomes the first stage in relaxation work. At this point, patients can be given the rationale of breath control as an important ingredient in relaxation.

The aim of this breath control method is to enable subjects to slow their breathing down by taking deep, steady, paced breaths as an aid to relaxation. Initially, provide an explanation of the interconnection of the respiratory and cardiovascular systems and the consequent speed with which the arousal level can be lowered by the introduction of paced, slow breathing. The difference between the breathing patterns of anxious and relaxed patients can be delineated, with emphasis placed on the difference between high, fast, short breaths that occur in anxiety (leading to all the symptoms of hyperventilation, etc.) and the slow, rhythmic, deep breathing of people when they are deeply relaxed. It should be pointed out that as the diaphragm contracts, the lungs can fill more deeply, and thus the rate of breathing can slow and the breaths become long and steady.

To teach diaphragmatic breathing, it is easiest to begin with the subjects lying flat on a couch or the floor so that they can place their hands on their midriffs and feel the changes that result from the intake of breath deep into the lungs. If the therapist can demonstrate the diaphragmatic breath, it will effectively aid training. Demonstrate the swelling of the midriff as the air comes in and the falling back of this part of the body and the rising of the chest as the breath is taken in completely. As the breath flows out, there is a drop in the chest and a full expiration occurs. Tightening in the chest reduces the scope of inflation of the lungs and leads to high, panting breaths. Encourage members of the group to define the characteristics of the demonstrated diaphragmatic breathing (even and long breaths, initial swelling of the abdomen, and rising of chest only at the end of respiration). Remind patients that when in pain (or anxious), breathing patterns are fast, shallow, and high in the chest. The latter can become habitual, especially when pain persists for years.

Patients should watch the therapist and then practice, preferably lying flat on the floor, couch, or bed where they can feel the effect in the midriff of deep inhalation and the contraction of the diaphragm. Group training is feasible as long as sessions can be held in a room large enough to allow the members of the group to lie flat on the floor during this practice period. If necessary, this breathing practice can be done seated, but it is more easily learned, initially, in a supine position, with hands placed on the midriff (fingertips touching at the midline) to gain feedback as to the depth of the breath. Ask patients to exhale, ridding themselves of all the air in their lungs. Ask them to inhale, directing the air down to their hands or to their midriff. This helps them take a large, deep breath and counteracts the tendency to panting, small, upper chest breathing. Once the cycle of intake and outflow of air has been established, encourage patients to make the two parts of the cycle equal and prolonged. In addition, encourage them to accentuate the swelling of the midriff at the onset of breath; this can, in fact, only be done by relaxation of the midriff and contraction of the diaphragm. By placing the hands parallel to the floor with fingertips touching (positioned over the midriff) they can see the fingers move away from each other as the air fills the lungs.

This method of breathing is a skill that is sometimes difficult for patients to learn, especially if they are tense in sessions, have a long history of smoking, have a tendency to hyperventilate, or are subject to chest and stomach tension. However, with practice, most patients can learn this method and find it beneficial in quickly inducing relaxation and in calming themselves. The long outbreath, which is established with training, allows them to concentrate their attention on relaxation of the muscles over a longer period of time and in itself becomes a cue that is used toward the end of this treatment as a strategy in pain management. "As you breathe out, let all the tension drain away from your body."

Problem Solving

Learning to control breathing may lead to the following problems:

- Patients sometimes feel the need to keep up a regular cycle of breathing without any prolonged intercycle interval. In fact, when a person becomes relaxed, he or she needs to breathe much less frequently, especially as the efficiency of each intake of air improves. Patients should be reminded of this, so that they do not feel any pressure to keep up a certain pace and can allow the frequency for these cycles to decrease.
- On taking in breaths at the onset, many patients will show a staccato intake pattern that probably relates to tension in the chest, thus preventing the easy expansion of the lungs. With reassurance and further relaxation of the upper chest, this will gradually be reduced, and they will be able to get a steady intake of air as they relax the chest.

- Some patients find themselves not filling their lungs sufficiently and wanting to take a number of small, panting breaths between cycles. Discourage this whenever possible, encouraging them to get used to utilizing each breath fully and thus inhibiting short, panting breaths.

- Some patients find the learning of this type of breathing tricky and may need reassurance that it is merely a matter of practice. Initially, practicing while sitting is always more difficult than when lying down. Once they have learned the technique lying down, they can resume a seated posture. Occasionally, there are some patients who seem unable to do this type of breathing. In such cases, emphasis should be on slow and regular breathing.

- Patients who smoke may find it more difficult to learn and may need to begin with shorter cycles, which they gradually lengthen.

- Aids to concentration on this type of breath control are useful if the patient is distractible or dealing with high levels of pain. In such a case, the patient is told to count slowly in each cycle (in-and-out equaling one cycle) in the following manner: (1) IN=2, 3, 4, OUT=2, 3, 4; (2) IN=2, 3, 4, OUT=2, 3, 4; (3) IN=2, 3, 4, OUT=2, 3, 4; (4) IN=2, 3, 4, OUT=2, 3, 4; . . . (10) IN=2, 3, 4, OUT=2, 3, 4. This ensures that the IN and OUT cycles are approximately the same length and can be speeded up or slowed down to meet the patient's own breathing pattern. It also encourages patients to do a full set of ten cycles while practicing.

It is wise to warn patients that, at the beginning, the increased intake of oxygen can make them feel a bit dizzy and lightheaded but that this is merely an effect of increasing the oxygen intake and will subside with further practice. It is, in fact, a sign that they are beginning to breathe more efficiently, and can be interpreted as a positive indication of progress.

HOMEWORK ASSIGNMENTS

Diaphragmatic Breathing

Firstly, the therapist should describe the assignments and directly relate them to the practical work undertaken. (Each patient may wish to keep an assignment book.) On this occasion, it is the practice of deep, slow, regular breathing, ten cycles on each occasion (in-and-out equaling one cycle), to be practiced on two separate occasions during each day, preferably lying down on a bed or floor in order to get the maximum training effect.

Exercise Monitoring

Secondly, for the next session, patients are asked to monitor exercise daily in order to establish an onset, or *base*, level. They are asked to select any one of three exercises (walking, bicycling, or swimming) and merely monitor how much they do, without changing their usual and characteristic exercise patterns. If patients are not undertaking any regular exercises, they are requested to put a 0 in each box on the monitoring sheets (see Appendix VIII). It is important to explain to patients that the aim is to clarify just what they are capable of doing during the first week. A sudden increase in order to make an entry on the sheet may produce discouraging after-effects. Emphasize this by pointing out to them that if they start at a low level, they can only increase and improve! In addition to monitoring a general exercise level, any specific exercises that they might be doing for their pain problem are to be monitored. They are asked to indicate the number of times they do them and to indicate in the lower grid which exercises they are undertaking (e.g., pelvic tilts: five times daily—see Appendix VI).

Pedometers worn for the first week may more accurately assess activity and exercise levels, though they will not clarify flexion exercise capacities. Exercise monitoring and use of a pedometer would allow the fullest evaluations.

Problem Solving

Patients often seem to have problems in understanding how to monitor their exercise; this can best be dealt with on the very first occasion of using the monitoring sheet with them. If there is any confusion in the group, fill in one on the blackboard in front of them to show them where they will be putting their numbers, running down the columns marked ''assess,'' starting from the day following the treatment session. Remind them to bring these back to all sessions.

SUGGESTED READINGS

Hawton, K., Salkovskis, P., Kirk, J., & Clark, D. (Eds.). (1989). *Cognitive behavior therapy for psychiatric problems.* Oxford: Oxford University Press.

Holzman, A., & Turk, D. (Eds.). (1986). *Pain management: A handbook of psychological treatment approaches.* NY: Pergamon Press.

Melzack, R., & Wall, P. (1988). *The challenge of pain.* Harmondsworth, UK: Penguin Books.

Pearce, S. (1983). A review of cognitive/behavioral methods for the treatment of chronic pain. *Journal of Psychosomatic Research, 27*(5), 431–440.

Weisenberg, M. (1987). Psychological intervention for the control of pain. *Behavior Research & Therapy, 25,* 301–312.

CHAPTER **8**

The Role of Relaxation
(Session #2)

REVIEW OF PREVIOUS ASSIGNMENTS

At the outset of this second session, allow time for discussion of any questions that may have arisen as a consequence of reading the handouts from the previous session and reflecting on the material raised.

Exercise Levels

It is important to establish the pattern of starting a session by reviewing homework assignments undertaken during the preceding week. In this session, the focus will be on the level of exercise that patients have monitored on their exercise sheets during the first week. From this the *average* amount of time spent walking (or swimming, etc.) can be estimated. Take one patient's monitoring sheet as an example and average it, showing the group how to total the number of minutes spent at the exercise and divide by seven to obtain the average level. Ask each person to exercise at their average level during the next week. For example, if a monitoring chart shows 20, 5, 0, 0, 10, 54, 5 minutes, the person would be asked to exercise for 94/7 = 14 minutes daily (see example sheet, Appendix VIII).

It is often the case that chronic pain patients have an off-and-on pattern of exercise, with periods of inactivity followed by a surge of exercise. The repercussions from the latter often lead to cessation of their activity patterns. This tendency needs to be broken during treatment, and a pattern of increasing exercise tolerance established. The best way to ensure success is to begin by setting the patient at a level well below the maximum he or she can achieve. In the example given earlier, a daily 14-minute exercise routine will seem very easy to achieve by a patient who, on some occasions, can go for as long as 54 minutes. They need to be encouraged to exercise at their average level for the next week, even though they may be keen to do more. Emphasize *daily* exercise at this relatively easy level, irrespective of pain levels. The average level will then be gradually increased as exercise tolerance increases, until the goal is reached.

In addition, discuss any problems that may have been met in breath control, resolving any difficulties that have arisen.

Goal Sheets

Finally, allow a short period of time to review the completed goal sheets. Family members may have offered some suggestions, and patients may wish to redefine, or make more precise, certain goals they have set for themselves that are unrealistic or insufficiently precise. With a group of six to eight people, it can be useful for the therapist to prepare specific goals for each person ahead of time. If such goals have not appeared on the patient's sheets, the therapist can try to persuade the person to add them. For example, a patient with a medication problem may need encouragement to include, in her last self-defined section, the following goal: "to reduce or eliminate my use of (pain) medications."

Problem Solving

At this stage, it is common for some members of the group to report that they have had no time or opportunity to undertake their homework. It is important to deal with this issue immediately. Make clear that the homework assignments are mandatory, being an *essential* part of the treatment approach. Skills are learned gradually by repeated practice, and the period between sessions allows this to be undertaken. Challenge the patients involved to complete omitted assignments by the next session. Make a point of asking them personally, at the beginning of the next session, whether they have managed to complete them. If necessary, solve problems that may have arisen with respect to family interference, lack of time alone, etc. Other members of the group can be encouraged to suggest ways in which the patient can overcome difficulties and arrange an exercise regime.

THE ROLE OF RELAXATION (TACTIC #lB)

The focus of the didactic presentation in this session is on the way in which relaxation can be used to modify or attenuate pain experience. As shown in Figure 7.3, p. 93, remind the group of the vicious cycle between pain and muscle tension. It is this cycle that the tactic of relaxation is designed to break.

The most common response to acute injury is to tighten the muscles, and this tightening acts to limit movement and promote healing. When pain becomes a chronic problem, the sufferer may develop permanent elevations in tension in certain muscles (e.g., masseter muscle, temporalis muscle, trapezius muscle). Unfortunately, this tensing and guarding, although often automatic muscular reactions to pain, can become habitual, unhelpful, and even counterproductive when pain becomes a chronic problem. The physical tension does not, in fact, reduce pain levels but is likely to increment or amplify the pain experienced.

Often, when this continues for many years, patients may lose awareness of how tense these muscles are. They may be unaware that areas around the pain locus are constantly tense, and it is only after relaxation skills are learned that the awareness of the overactivity of certain muscles grows.

The aim of the current session is to provide the background to the introduction of this major tactic—progressive relaxation. This type of relaxation is unlike the ordinary relaxation that most people feel when flopped in front of the television, or even when asleep. In this relaxation, the patient remains alert and in control. In addition, they will be concentrating, not merely on physical calmness and reduced muscle tension, but also upon emotional calmness, which can be induced by the learning of physical techniques to relax the muscles. The ultimate goal is for the people to be able to "turn on" a relaxation response within 3 to 5 minutes. When patients reach this level of skill, they can use relaxation induction as a specific tactic to manage difficult pain episodes (episodic control). Even without this degree of control, a longer, 20-minute induction (necessary at the onset of training) begins to teach the person the difference between tension and relaxation, so that a remarkable degree of calm can be gradually induced.

The capacity to relax at will is a complex skill. Some people report that they feel able to relax, although they may never have had any training and have no understanding of how to achieve it. Training is necessary across a number of weeks in order to learn this skill. It is for this reason that the relaxation tactic is introduced as early as possible in treatment, so that at least seven to eight weeks are available to concentrate on the development of this skill.

Relaxation techniques can be taught in various ways, and a useful method is the modification of the Bernstein and Borkovec (1973) method. This training in progressive relaxation systematically teaches the persons to relax the major muscle groups throughout the body. A progressive capacity to relax is taught in a graded and systematic manner, thus giving it the name of progressive or systematic relaxation. It is a well-established technique in clinical psychology, popularized by J. Wolpe (1958) drawing upon the work of Jacobson (1938). It has become a frequently used method of the behavior therapist, particularly with respect to the management of anxiety and phobias. A modified version of the Bernstein and Borkovec method can be used in pain groups. This allows training to be taught in a 20-minute period, with attention being focused on the following nine muscle groups in sequence: legs (two different exercises); arms; stomach and midriff; buttocks; thighs and pelvic floor; chest; shoulders; neck (two exercises); jaw and facial muscles. Therapists unfamiliar with this method are referred to the Bernstein and Borkovec manual for further details.

This method of training in relaxation utilizes a sequence of tensing prior to relaxation, in order to demonstrate the initial relaxation response. The person is encouraged to "read" the level of tension in a muscle group and learn the difference in kinesthetic feedback when tense and when relaxed. As they grow more aware of the sensation of tension in a particular muscle group, they can learn more readily to actively relax those muscles when they wish. As they progress, people become more aware of how tension can build up. They then begin to monitor and reduce this when it occurs during their usual activities.

Relaxation can be deepened by combining it with paced diaphragmatic breathing. The relaxation response is encouraged with the exhalation and release of tension, while tensing the muscle initially is combined with inhalation. Ultimately the exhalation can become an important and quick cue for invoking relaxation and is taught in Session #8, as the ninth training tactic. Cue relaxation cannot be undertaken until relaxation is well learned. However, from the beginning, the combination of the relaxation response with the exhalation establishes a conditioned association that can be utilized at a later stage.

A simple demonstration by the therapist of the effect of tensing prior to relaxing, will demonstrate to the group the reason for using this sequence during training. Alternatively, the patients themselves can be asked to first relax both arms into their laps and sit comfortably. When they feel they are as relaxed as possible, it is pointed out to them that there are areas of tension in their bodies that perhaps they had not been aware of (e.g., where their legs cross, where their arms rest, perhaps in the shoulders, at the base of the spine).

They are asked to relax both arms using any tactic they can. Then they are given instructions to relax the right arm by first tensing the biceps (for a count of 10) and then releasing the tension. Ask them to compare the right arm with the left arm, which has remained in their lap, and note any differences. Encourage the group to generate differences in sensation between the two arms (e.g., warmth, heaviness, tingling). These are useful clues that their muscles are relaxing.

Remind them at this stage that it is very important to work more cautiously when tensing muscles close to the pain locus. A slight increase above the usual level is all that is needed in order to gain the relaxation effect. Caution against an overzealous approach to this skill (e.g., with clenching the teeth in facial pain, shoulder exercises for those with shoulder injuries and upper quadrant problems). Spasms in unused muscles or consequent muscle soreness can lead to a novice withdrawing from training or refusing to practice this skill.

PROGRESSIVE RELAXATION (TACTIC #1C)

The tactic of progressive relaxation is now practiced by the group. Ask each patient to choose the most comfortable position in which to relax (lying or sitting). If some choose to lie down, ensure that back pain patients have their feet on the ground, close to the buttocks, with their knees up, and that neck pain patients have a roll or pillow underneath their neck. In some cases, they may find it more comfortable to sit on a hard-backed chair. For the majority, lying on the floor is probably the best option, because it allows them to notice their diaphragmatic breathing and to relax more easily at this early stage of skill learning.

Start by encouraging the group to begin deepening their breaths in order to establish regular, steady exchanges of air, preferably using the diaphragmatic method taught in the previous session. Once this has been established, begin working with the leg muscles, utilizing the two major exercises from the Bernstein and Borkovec method. Leg muscles are useful to begin with as they are quite easily relaxed by most people. In this initial induction, it may be wise to relax one leg at a time, thus allowing the patient to make comparisons between tension and relaxation states. Once patients have relaxed their legs, allow them a period of time just to enjoy the feeling of heaviness and relaxation of the legs, then move on to the other areas mentioned above. Focus the attention of particular people in the group on specific muscle groups that are relevant to their pain problem. For example, patients with neck and shoulder problems can be reminded of the importance of relaxing the trapezius and of allowing the shoulders to fall as low as possible (when you reach the exercises that relate to these muscles).

Monitor all the patients in your group continuously to ensure that they are following instructions and not running into any particular difficulties. This is not a difficult task to undertake, as long as the group does not exceed eight people. The majority of patients follow instructions well, although they may need reminders to keep using their deep breathing in association with the exercises. Problems may arise with certain patients when concentrating on muscles near the pain locus. The avoidance posture that is so often seen in chronic pain patients can be interestingly observed in their approach to these muscular exercises. Specific encouragement may well be necessary in patients who are tensing prior to the onset of certain exercises in anticipation of pain increment. Where there is a marked avoidance of an exercise, grade the person into the initial tensing in slow steps.

Problem Solving

The major difficulty in this session is dealing with patients who expect immediate results from the initial session of relaxation and are frustrated by their inability to achieve it instantly. The aim is to begin to reinforce the idea of *skill development*. Remind impatient people of learning to ride a bicycle, or other skills which increase with practice.

The specification of a particular time to practice relaxation is often very important, as homework assignments can be sabotaged by patient or family. Compliance is improved if patients can gain agreement from their families about when they can be alone to work on this skill.

HOMEWORK ASSIGNMENTS

Practice

Regular practice of the relaxation method demonstrated is essential if the skill is to be perfected. Once this is achieved, patients will have at their command the skill to significantly reduce the pain experience within minutes, a skill they can call upon when and if they need it. At this stage, prescribe two practices daily for a full 20 minutes at a time, working systematically through the nine muscle groups. Patients need to be encouraged to find a particular time of the day when they will do this work. Seeking help from their spouse or partner may ensure that they can have two 20-minute periods to undertake this assignment. Concentration and compliance can be increased by providing taped relaxation instructions.

Preparation for Session #3

Preparation for the next session is threefold. First, physical exercise (walking, swimming, or exercise bicycling) at the average time level established during the first week's monitoring is to begin on a *daily* basis. Proof of consistent daily exercise at the initial (basal) level is required prior to any increments. If performance was erratic during the first week, challenge patients to begin consistent daily exercise regimes, at a certain time of day, for the average time period established (e.g., 5 minutes of walking daily—2.5 minutes in one direction, and 2.5 minutes on the return trip).

Second, ask the members of the group to begin keeping an accurate account of the variations in their pain problems. Provide them with monitoring booklets similar to those used in the pretreatment assessment. This will allow them to begin systematically to analyze the variations in their pain problem, the factors influencing it, and the effects of various tactics that are being introduced. When pain continues for many years, this kind of information often becomes blurred and unclear, and the person's memory is filled with the worst and most upsetting moments of the day, which are remembered as having been interminably long. As they begin to monitor their own pain problems over a few weeks, they become more aware of the variability of the pain experience. As a homework assignment, ask them to monitor their pain levels hourly for the seven days until they return, looking for the following characteristics of their own pain problem:

1. How constant is the pain (i.e., how long does it remain at the same level during the day)? If there is any variation in the intensity of the pain, this implies that it is having a variable influence on the patient's life and is in fact *not* continuous, everlasting, and negative.
2. Ask them to clarify how often the pain level remains stable despite the fact that they have undertaken activities. Any occasion when this occurs will illustrate that it is *not always* worsened by activity undertaken. On some occasions, they may even be able to detect stability or even reductions in pain level while undertaking work, when busy talking to friends, or when engaging in a pleasant activity.
3. They should also be encouraged to look out for patterns in their pain levels, thus increasing its predictability. They may notice

that it tends to increase during the day, to peak at mealtimes, to be much more intense on waking, when quarreling with friends or relations, under arousing conditions, and so forth. They may notice that it is much worse if they push themselves to do more than they are capable of achieving. A rebound may occur during or after the activity.

4. Encourage them to notice how long the worst levels of pain last. Perhaps they can be encouraged to give an average time during which they experience the highest level of pain. This will illustrate to them that these difficult periods are relatively transitory and always reduce to a lower level at some point.

5. Ask them to predict and record the peak pain level they *expect* during their major daily exercise, and then compare this prerecorded prediction with the actual peak pain experienced during the exercise.

Overall, the therapist should make the point that the sense of hopelessness and endless suffering that is often felt by chronic pain patients needs to be reevaluated in light of the variability that can be found in their own pain records. Periods of intense pain are always followed by reductions to more manageable levels, and the initial tendency to overpredict their pain levels gradually subsides as they become increasingly accurate in their predictions.

The reason for undertaking this self-examination of pain levels is that people will be in a much better position to manage their pain problems using the tactics they are taught. During the circumscribed periods of intense pain, patients will be able to call upon specific behavioral and cognitive tactics that they have learned. The difficult periods last only for a relatively short time. The aim is to keep the pain under control and to keep it manageable by using the techniques learned. The more patients understand about their own pain patterns and how to affect them, the better able they will be to modulate the pain levels and lessen the impact on their lives.

The therapist, at this stage, is encouraging patients to be private investigators, finding out as much as can be learned about the characteristics of the pain problem. The more predictable and understandable their difficulties, the easier it will be to gain control over them.

The booklets allow each person to monitor systematically. A small instruction leaflet can be provided to remind patients about the hourly marking of the booklet and the circling of the hour at which they went to bed and woke up. Such a leaflet will save the therapist time. Request that monitoring be undertaken for the next week and that the booklets be brought back at the next session.

Finally, in preparation for the analgesic reduction program for those with medication dependence (Session #4), patients are requested at this time to take their medications three to four times daily, judging by the clock rather than by pain levels. They are asked to use whatever medications they are currently on, divided into three or four doses, as a prelude to the graded reduction program.

The reason for this change is explained in detail in Session #4.

SUGGESTED READINGS

Bernstein, D. A., & Borkovec, T. D. (1973). *Progressive relaxation training: A manual for helping professions.* Champaign, IL: Research Press.

Jacobson, E. (1938). *Progressive relaxation.* Chicago: Chicago University Press.

Lichstein, K. (1988). *Clinical relaxation strategies.* New York: Wiley.

Linton, S. J. (1982). Applied relaxation as a method of coping with chronic pain—A therapist's guide. *The Scandinavian Journal of Behavior Therapy, 11,* 161–174.

Turner, J., & Chapman, C. R. (1982). Psychological interventions for chronic pain: A critical review, I and II. *Pain, 12,* 1–46.

Wolpe, J. (1958). *Psychotherapy by reciprocal inhibition.* Stanford, CA: Stanford University Press.

CHAPTER 9

The Role of Exercise
(Session #3)

REVIEW OF PREVIOUS ASSIGNMENTS

By beginning the session with a discussion of previous assignments, the
therapist directs the attention of the group to what they have been able
to achieve as opposed to how much pain they have been experiencing.
Elicit the extent to which the members of the group have practiced relaxation, undertaken daily exercise, and used their analgesics on a time-
linked basis. Encourage the poor compliers to follow the group example,
giving them specific challenges. Keeping a checklist of compliance with
assignments can be useful for the therapist; acting as a reminder of progress
made by members of the group (see Appendix IV).

Self-Monitoring Results

Most of the first part of this session can usefully be used in a discussion
of the conclusions that each patient has drawn about his or her pain pattern
as a consequence of self-monitoring. Try to use particular examples, taken

from patients' pain diaries, to illustrate the peaks and troughs in patterns, drawing out the implications with respect to the varying influence of pain on the patients. At its lowest levels (when the pain is at level 0, 1, or 2), pain can be endured and may not interfere with ongoing activities. At higher levels (at 4 and 5 in intensity) the pain may interrupt activities and concentration. At such times, active coping tactics are needed in order to continue despite pain. These tactics are to be taught during sessions and are best practiced, initially, when patients are experiencing lower levels of pain. As the pain reaches high levels, it is more difficult to control and requires a higher level of skill and experience with the tactics.

Point out that pain levels may remain stable during many activities undertaken during the week and that pain intensity will not inevitably increase. In some cases, the therapist can point out occasions when changes in activities or increasing activities actually *reduced* pain levels for a person. Make sure to point out that the worst levels of pain do not last indefinitely and are, in fact, relatively transient. Encourage members of the group to average or form an estimate of the number of minutes or hours that they usually suffer their worst episodes. Emphasis on the peaking nature of bad episodes leads patients to realize that only a short period of management is needed in order to pass through these bad periods.

Some patients may begin to notice patterns in their pain problems associated with certain stimuli (e.g., worrying, rushing, exercising, quarreling). The therapist's aim during this discussion is to encourage each member of the group to begin to analyze the pattern of his or her pain problem so that it becomes predictable and the coping tactics can be used effectively. The greater the capacity of each person to predict pain levels, the greater his or her sense of control. The repeated exercise of predicting peak pain levels and then checking the accuracy of the prediction enables patients to improve their ability to anticipate painful and pain-free episodes.

THE ROLE OF EXERCISE

The didactic presentation in this session draws out the consequences of disuse and inactivity upon chronic pain. The benefits of increasing activity tolerance and fitness are described. Finally, the way in which the habits of inactivity and withdrawal can be counteracted is discussed in detail, and an activity program suggested to the group.

The Effects of Disuse and Inactivity

When a person sustains an acute injury, it takes a certain number of days or weeks for the tissue to heal. We now know that injuries to the skin will take approximately one to two days to two weeks to heal, and six to seven weeks until the injured limb returns to full strength. Muscles and soft tissue take from one to three weeks to heal and approximately seven to twelve weeks to return to full strength. Fractures take four to six weeks to heal and six months to one year to completely mend. Finally, complex joint fractures can take three to four months to heal and up to one year to return to normal.

In other words, the healing time for different types of injury is relatively short, after which time scar tissue forms and there is no longer any physical evidence of acute injury. As healing is completed, the person will gradually resume use of the injured limb or muscle group.

When pain continues past the healing of soft tissue, muscle, or ligament, there is a tendency for the sufferer to continue resting and remain inactive, as if these responses might resolve the pain problem. Unfortunately, the brain seems unable to distinguish between the messages that come to it from recently injured tissue and those that come from residual scarring, straining of inflexible and tight muscles, postural adaptations to continuing pain, and so forth. These messages may become the physical signals received by the brain that are interpreted as "pain . . . danger . . . tissue damage . . . " Although this may be appropriate for the acutely injured person, it is not helpful to the chronic pain sufferer. Inactivity and rest become less and less useful during the recuperative period. In the case of a chronic pain problem, when healing is complete, the recuperative period is over. It has been found that continuing disuse may in fact make the problem worse and contribute to the development of "invalid status" (Fordyce, Brockway, Bergman, & Spingler, 1985).

There are at least three major reasons why inactivity and withdrawal may exacerbate a chronic pain problem. The more inactive the person becomes, the weaker and less flexible the muscles become. As a consequence, when physical demands are made upon these muscles, they become strained and fatigued by the slightest movement. The sensations confirm to the sufferer that he or she should remain inactive because the damage or disturbance of tissue remains. This leads to a spiraling vicious cycle, as illustrated in Figure 7.3, p. 93. It is, of course, not surprising that inactivity will lead to discomfort and pain. It has been estimated that within one week of total immobility, a muscle loses approximately one-third of its size and power. One has merely to look at the limb following the removal of a cast to recognize the magnitude of these changes. Six weeks of an arm being held immobile by a sling (with no previous injury) produce the same muscular symptoms as those produced in a person who has had his or her limb in a cast due to a previous break. It has been estimated that 30% demineralization of the bone occurs after only two weeks of bed rest, and that this is not completely repaired for up to 10 years! The one week's complete bed rest, so often prescribed for back pain problems, can lead to a rapid reduction in muscular strength. It is important to draw out these consequences of inactivity for chronic pain patients so that they begin to realize that the tendency to remain inactive—which seems so appropriate to the pain patients themselves—is, in fact, an important element in sustaining and even increasing the problem (Boltz, 1984).

With reduced activity and withdrawal from any physical activity, sufferers become increasingly helpless and may feel defeated by their problem. They are unable to undertake activities that have been rewarding and enjoyable to them. Their lowered mood may lead to the development of another vicious cycle between depression and pain tolerance. Cut off from stimulation, the sensations from the body are probably heightened in the awareness of sufferers. Nothing distracts them from detecting, weighing, and evaluating every feeling and sensation that comes from their bodies. It is not surprising, therefore, to find chronic pain sufferers preoccupied with the pain sensation and all the factors that can exacerbate it.

Much less well researched, but of considerable interest in pain management, is the fact that exercise appears to activate the body's own natural defense system. In the last few years, physiologists have studied the natural morphine-like substance known as endorphin, which many patients will have read about in the lay press. It is produced in the brain and acts to block the transmission of electrical signals between the nerve cells carrying pain messages. When endorphin levels are high, the pain experience is reduced. High levels of endorphin have been found in athletes, helping to explain why they are capable of enduring long periods of exertion. In contrast, endorphin levels are low in chronic pain sufferers. It seems possible that increasing activity level may start to boost a person's production of endorphins. These notions are relatively new and have not been fully evaluated to date. However, they are worth discussing with patients and provide an additional motivation for engaging in an exercise program that many of them may feel reluctant to undertake initially.

The Normality of Inactivity as a Reaction to Pain

Irrespective of the locus or chronicity of the pain problem, the majority of chronic pain patients appear to have reacted to the continual aversive pain experience by inactivity, thus losing fitness. The vicious cycles described above lead to the maintenance of this pattern of behavior, even when pain levels are low. Anticipatory avoidance of exercise and activity may be present because of a mounting fear that the pain problem will get worse if they return to a more normal life. Avoidance patterns appear to be less common in headache sufferers, who may develop a tendency to become overactive, broken by periods of complete inactivity. When such a cycle occurs, there is less disuse, and often they remain physically fit.

The Benefits of Increasing Activity Tolerance and Fitness

As an encouragement to patients who are reluctant to engage in physical activity, it is important to delineate the benefits that ensue from such a regimen. They can look forward to strengthening the muscles and increasing flexibility. They will also gain stamina as they become more tolerant of exercise.

From a psychological point of view, the activity program can be a potent method of gradually discrediting a strong belief that develops in many chronic pain patients. They grow to believe that any increase in physical activity will necessarily lead to pain provocation (they overpredict the pain), with the possibility of becoming permanent invalids. It is important that this belief be challenged, and the graded exercise program acts in a systematic way to break down the assumption of fragility. The exercise program increases physical stamina and strengthens muscles and also invalidates the belief that any activity, other than the most minimal routine, will lead to disastrous effects with respect to future mobility, pain, and ill-health.

In addition, an increasing sense of well-being and elevation in mood often result when exercise is introduced for chronic pain patients. To what extent this has anything to do with the release of endorphins is unclear. However, patients often report that they begin to feel their spirits rise as a consequence of having completed their exercise program each day, and documented reduction in depression as a consequence of treatment (Philips, 1987a) may relate, in part, to the use of an active exercise component.

Instigating the Exercise Regime

The practical issue of how to break the vicious cycles described previously leads to the description of the way in which to develop a personal exercise program. It is important to emphasize that physical activity will be encouraged in a gradual manner. It is essential to work slowly and steadily toward a goal that may, at the onset, seem impossible. The initial steps are small, but as such they are more likely to be complied with and lead to success when quotas are met. Setting the initial exercise levels slightly below the average makes it likely that the patient will continue his or her exercise irrespective of current pain levels, thus meeting the therapist's requests. The attempt is to break through a well-established off-and-on pattern of activity, in which the patient may try some exercises at an extreme level, suffer pain repercussions, and give it up entirely. After a period of inactivity, the patient may repeat this overactivity, followed by defeat. It is this on-and-off pattern of activity that can become an important exacerbator of the whole chronic pain cycle. (This issue is dealt with in detail in Session #8.)

Requesting very gradual increases in exercise endurance shows the patients that they can gradually raise their exercise levels by graded and gradual changes so as not to produce repercussions. Examples of overactivity and its consequences are often available from members of the group or can be interjected as examples by the therapist (e.g., a person who does not exercise for three months and then decides to dig up the vegetable patch, or the person who starts to exercise for the first time by jogging for 50 minutes up a hill).

It is important to emphasize from the onset that a regular exercise program is one that is undertaken daily. This being the case, the goal for each day must be realistic and feasible, given the person's daily routine and extent of pain. Two types of exercise can be encouraged:

1. General exercise can be obtained through walking, swimming, or biking. These exercises are appropriate for virtually any chronic pain patient, although a brisk walking routine is often the easiest to implement, being independent of the availability of facilities. Try to get patients to nominate the exercises of their choice, which they will then undertake throughout the program. Patients wishing to undertake all three, or two of these types of exercise, can be encouraged to arrange such a program.

   Advise the patients from the onset that their exercise will be on a daily basis. With onset levels set low, no strain will be produced. No time pressure should be put on the activity initially, and walking up hills or using weighted pedals on bicycles should be discouraged at the beginning.

   If a physical therapist is not available to advise the therapist on an appropriate general exercise goal, encourage patients to work toward a daily exercise average of 20 to 30 minutes of brisk exercise. For some patients, this may require a gradual process of building up the length of time they can exercise until they reach the goal. For others, it may be a question of breaking the on-and-off pattern of exercise and obtaining a commitment to regular (daily) general exercise.

2. If possible, it is useful to encourage patients to undertake a set of special flexion exercises to strengthen muscle groups that have become weak and inactive. If available, a consultant physical therapist may be willing to provide personally tailored flexion exercise programs for each patient in the group. These can be undertaken in a gradually incrementing manner as part of the general exercise program.

If no physical therapist is available to coordinate with the therapy program, a set of flexion exercises, which will help improve posture or strengthen the weakened, disused muscles, can be utilized. A set of simple exercises that are useful for chronic pain patients is provided in Appendix II.

Why Increased Exercise is Encouraged
From the Beginning of the Program

Starting from the outset with this approach to exercise establishes and encourages the proper participation of members of the group. The psychological effect of the gradual increase in exercise is valuable from the onset of treatment. Changes can be seen in this capacity much more quickly than in some of the complex control skills, which can be taught later in the treatment program. In addition, this tactic, like progressive relaxation, needs considerable practice and encouragement over as many weeks as possible. Starting the activity program in the third week gives the patients at least six weeks of treatment to establish their exercise program. For the majority of people, this proves sufficient to reach the suggested goal levels for both general exercise and for flexion exercises.

GRADED EXERCISE (TACTIC #2)

The practical section of this session is spent in explaining, demonstrating, and practicing specific exercises that patients can use to gain increasing flexibility and power in the key areas weakened because of injury or pain. In addition, the general exercise program (walking, swimming, or bicycling) can be further clarified for patients, and any problems resolved in this respect. The specific daily increments to be undertaken by pain patients need to be reviewed so that they appreciate the rate of increment that is required of them.

More specific flexion exercises can be demonstrated in the session. If no physical therapist is available to advise on each patient's needs, choose a group of exercises from Appendix II, keeping in mind the pain locus and weakened muscles. Head pain sufferers may be best aided by undertaking the exercises in Sections 1 (a to c) and 5. Remember to encourage patients to start at a very low level and to gradually increase up to 10 repetitions per day. Those exercises marked with an * are particularly useful for patients with mid- and lower-back problems. However, none of the exercises, if done in a gradual manner, will be anything but beneficial for chronic pain problems.

Problem Solving

The major difficulty a therapist will encounter in establishing a regular exercise program is with lack of adherence. It is hard for pain patients to believe that engaging in an activity program (which may in the past have led to increasing pain) can be a useful tactic for gradually bringing the problem under their own control. A number of different methods can be used to improve adherence to the program.

1. The self-monitoring of exercise over a number of weeks often is a useful method of providing the patient with positive indications that he or she is gradually increasing his or her exercise without producing deleterious results. (An example of such an instrument for the monitoring of exercise is given in Appendix VIII.)
2. Many pain patients find that the introduction of an exercise program is difficult to undertake because of the disruption it may cause in other aspects of their lives (e.g., having time on their own, resentments of spouse or family about their absence while exercising). These effects are usefully discussed with patients, as they often raise other issues concerning patients' rights in their family; their ability to assert their needs, to pace their time, and so forth. Initially, encourage patients to discuss the exercise program with spouse or partner, and even involve them in it. A friend may be persuaded to join the exercise program with them. Exercise compliance rates will be higher with the involvement of a partner. However patients start at a much lower level than those without a chronic pain problem, and, in the early stages, they may need to exercise alone.
3. Graphing progress at the onset can be an aid to patients who are having adherence problems.

HOMEWORK ASSIGNMENTS

Exercise

Ask patients to begin exercising on a daily basis, starting from levels well below their capacity when feeling at best (e.g., slightly below their average exercise time) and gradually increasing week by week toward a 30-minute brisk walk, swim, or bike ride by the end of treatment. If a physical therapist is available, he or she may be able to give advice on the appropriate incremental rate. If such advice is not available, use a gradual increase initially, making larger demands as the person's confidence grows with respect to reaching weekly goals. Often patients overestimate what they will be able to do, and it is best to set easily achieved goals at this stage in order to keep up their confidence in their capacity to exercise. Patients who, for example, have shown in their basal recordings that they are able to manage a daily average of five minutes of walking might be encouraged to raise this for the next week to eight minutes a day. The response to this increment will guide the therapist on the size of the next increment. Emphasis should be placed on regular exercise, whatever the level and whatever the weather.

Begin all specific exercises at one to two cycles per day, gradually increasing the demand over the weeks until patients have reached ten cycles one to two times daily. If they find they can and wish to do more, encourage this to be done on a gradual, incremental basis. Where a physical therapist is available, he or she may suggest alternative goals for specific persons. As a therapist, initially err on the side of caution in demands made of patients. Once the first few weeks have brought success, steadily and persistently increase the demands on performance at each exercise period.

Drug Intake

In preparation for a discussion on the role of drugs and the beginning of analgesic reduction programs, patients should be asked to move onto a liquid equivalent of their current drug intake. Explain this step to them insuring that they understand that an exact liquid equivalent of their usual drug dose is being prescribed to be taken at regular times in the day (three to four times daily). This will produce no change, but it is the first step in facilitating reduction in subsequent sessions. It may be useful to provide a handout to patients about the drug reduction approach, so that they are fully cognizant of what will be involved. Reassure them that the next session will give them ample opportunity to discuss these issues and that no reduction in their medication will be undertaken without their knowledge. It is sometimes the case that when patients are moved across to a time-based medication regimen, pain levels drop slightly. Changes in drug taking, however, may be met with considerable anxiety, and the therapist should leave time in this session for giving adequate reassurance to those patients who are taking this step toward a graded reduction of their dependency.

Pain Diary

Ask patients to fill in their pain diaries for another week and ask them to watch carefully for any patterns that may emerge as a consequence of a change of activity and the introduction of the exercise program, as well as the change to a time-based drug regimen.

Relaxation Practice

Remind patients again to continue using their relaxation tapes twice daily so that the skill of muscular relaxation can be well learned. Remind them that during the next session, time will be allowed to check on their progress.

SUGGESTED READINGS

Boltz, W. (1984). The disuse syndrome. *Western Journal of Medicine, 141*, 691–694.

Doleys, D. M., Crocker, M., & Pattoen, B. (1982). Responses of patients with chronic pain to exercise quotas. *Journal of the American Physiotherapy Association, 62*(8), 111–114.

Fordyce, W. E., Brockway, J., Bergman, J., & Spingler, D. (1985). Acute back pain: A control group comparison of behavioral and traditional management methods. *Journal of Behavioral Medicine, 9*(2), 127–140.

Linton, S. J. (1985). Relationship between activity and chronic back pain. *Pain, 21*, 289–294.

Meichenbaun, D., & Turk, D. (1990). *Facilitating treatment adherence.* New York: Plenum Press.

CHAPTER 10

The Role of Drugs
(Session #4)

REVIEW OF PREVIOUS ASSIGNMENTS

Begin by eliciting the reactions of the group to the increases in their exercise program, to the move to liquid analgesics, and to the use of tapes to attain rapid and deep relaxation.

Problem Solving

Exercise Regime

Patients who had difficulties in keeping up with their exercise goals for the week may need to have an additional week to achieve them. Exercise levels can be maintained at their current level at any point during treatment, but it is unwise to drop back unless absolutely necessary. If the basal level is set appropriately, and incrementing quotas are small and gradual, there should be no reason to drop back unless some unforeseen circumstance occurs (e.g., the patient falls or becomes ill). Maintenance at the previous week's level is the best way to deal with reports of difficulty.

It has the added benefit of making the patient feel in control of the pacing of his or her program.

Drug Reduction

Some patients react negatively to the shift to the liquid analgesic even though no pharmacological change has occurred. It may take a few days for them to settle into the regime. In this case, the first reduction can be delayed a week while they maintain 100% liquid equivalent for another week. Again, their anxieties about loss of control are addressed.

Most of the initial period of this session will be usefully spent looking again at the self-monitoring diaries of the patients in the group. For those who have not contributed to this discussion in the previous weeks, encourage the clarification of individual pain patterns that they may be able to associate with certain situations or stimuli.

THE ROLE OF DRUGS

The aim of this session is to make the patients minor experts on the nature of drugs used for the management of chronic pain, their actions, and their limitations. The discussion will need to be simplified in order to make it readily understandable, and attempts should be made by the therapist to keep it as factual as possible. Trade names of drugs are useful to patients, as they learn the nature of their medication and the side-effects. Wherever possible, try to include the consultant pharmacist in this session, either by making a presentation or by joining in the discussion for this portion of the session. Additional weight is thus given to the discussion, especially as the dependency of individual patients can be used as illustrative material by the pharmacist (who has assessed each person prior to the onset of the group). The pharmacist also helps in re-education about drug constituents, actions and side-effects.

The Usefulness of Drugs for Pain Management

It is commonly believed that chemical intervention is the treatment of choice for pain control. Such medications are generally very effective in short-term use for acute pain, but unfortunately they have been found to lose their effectiveness and become of questionable value in the management of chronic, persisting pain. Paradoxically, as their efficacy in reducing the pain decreases, their side-effects sometimes increase, as do the physiological and psychological dependencies of the user. In conditions such as rheumatoid arthritis and cancer pain, chronic analgesic use may be required. However, for many people with chronic, benign pain problems, the pain/medication interaction can become a vicious circle, with the pain becoming increasingly difficult to manage. When the effectiveness of the medication decreases and the side-effects become annoying or uncomfortable, it is time for the patient to re-evaluate the situation and find alternative methods for managing the chronic pain.

Types of Drugs and Their Side-Effects

An overview is provided below of the major types of drugs used in the management of chronic pain: peripherally acting analgesics (aspirin, acetaminophen), centrally acting analgesics (narcotics), adjuvant analgesics (barbiturates, antidepressants, tranquilizers, and anxiolytics), and muscular relaxants. Finally, drugs specifically designed for a particular pain problem (e.g., antimigraine drugs) are included.

Peripherally Acting Analgesics

The three major analgesics of this type are aspirin (i.e., acetylsalicylic acid, or ASA); acetaminophen (e.g., Tylenol®, Exdol®, Atasol®); and other nonsteroidal anti-inflammatory drugs (NSAIDs) (Motrin®, Nuprin®, Indocin®, Naprosyn®, Dolobid®).[1]

Unlike centrally acting analgesics, these drugs have not been found to be associated with physical dependencies, addiction, or adverse side-effects, but toxic effects are possible with excessive use. In addition, psychological dependencies can develop despite the unpleasant side-effects. The drugs appear to inhibit the synthesis of prostaglandin, a substance that sensitizes free nerve endings to the algogenic substance, bradykinin. In addition, aspirin has an anti-inflammatory effect.

---

[1]Trademark symbols will be listed at first mention only.

The side-effects of aspirin can include abdominal pain, nausea, tinnitus, and respiratory problems in those prone to allergic reactions. However, it should be pointed out that dangerous side-effects occur in only 15% of those taking aspirin (Aronoff & Wagner, 1986). Although patients may develop a pattern of taking increasing amounts of aspirin, therapeutic improvement will not follow from increasing the dose beyond approximately 1,000 mg every four hours (Aronoff, Evans, & Enders, 1985).

Acetaminophen does not have anti-inflammatory properties, but in other respects has the same effects as aspirin. In addition, it does not have any adverse side-effects with respect to gastrointestinal function.

NSAIDs do not appear to have any major advantages that cannot be achieved through aspirin use and have varied side-effects, depending on the choice of drugs.

Centrally Acting Analgesics

These act on the central nervous system by binding to opiate receptor sites and activating an endogenous pain modulation system (Aronoff, Wagner, & Spangler, 1986). These drugs are classed as narcotics and are either natural or synthetic derivatives of morphine or opium. Some common examples are: codeine (Tylenol® #2, 3, 4); Frosst® 292, 222; meperidine (Demerol®); pentazocine (Talwin®); morphine; oxycodone (Percodan®, Percocet®); propoxyphene (Darvon®, Frosst® 692).

Unfortunately, there are a number of important and problematic consequences of repeated use of these drugs. An unavoidable consequence of protracted use of these drugs (which of course will occur with a chronic pain problem) is the *growth of tolerance*. The doses become progressively less effective, and larger doses become necessary to achieve any analgesic effect. The two consequences of this growing tolerance are an increase in side-effects and physical dependency. The latter takes the form of withdrawal symptoms if the narcotic medication is stopped. Because of the depressant effects of these drugs on the central nervous system, side-effects such as constipation, nausea, vomiting, decreased lung function, sleep disturbance, headaches, dizziness, light-headedness, and depression/elation can be produced. Slowed reaction time, mental confusion, and impairment of new learning may also occur. Because the narcotic can produce euphoria, at least immediately after ingestion, chronic pain patients with mood difficulties may become dependent upon this lift or "high" from the intake of their drugs. The withdrawal of these drugs when this pattern has arisen becomes a more complex issue.

In an attempt to overcome the side-effects of these drugs, synthetic compounds have been developed. Combinations of aspirin, acetaminophen, and caffeine have been produced (Tylenol® #3, Frosst 292, Exdol 30, Atasol 30, Percodan, and Percocet). It has been calculated that the caffeine included in one Frosst 292 is equivalent to two cups of black coffee. Caffeine is introduced to counteract the drowsiness produced by the narcotic. Unfortunately, the predicted benefits often do not continue with chronic use of the medication. In addition, for some people with vascular headaches, the caffeine can increase their headache frequency. The caffeine causes overexcitation, sometimes making sleep difficult and increasing agitation. This occurs because of the longer action of caffeine (seven hours to half effect) than of codeine (three hours to half effect).

To counteract the overexcitation produced by caffeine, synthetic compounds have been produced that combine aspirin, codeine, caffeine, and butalbital (a barbiturate used in sleeping drugs). A common example of this combination of drugs is Fiorinal® C1/2. This product provides some pain relief, but may also increase the side-effects, binding the many problems of each of the component drugs into one capsule. In this case, the combination is to speed up *and* to make the person sleep. It is difficult to wean patients from these drugs once psychological and physiological dependence is present. The withdrawal process needs to be done with great care and in a structured, graded manner. If a patient has a physiological dependence upon narcotics, it is unwise to undertake the graded reduction without the advice and collaboration of a pharmacist.

Adjuvant Analgesics

The third group of analgesics are called "adjuvant analgesics" by Foley (1985), even though the analgesic value of such medications is unclear. There are many different types of drugs that can be considered in this category, but perhaps the most important are the tranquilizers (sedatives, hypnotics, and anti-anxiety medications). An example of these types of drugs are barbiturates, diazepam (Valium®), oxazepam (Serax®), lorazepam (Ativan®), alprazolam (Xanax®), and flurazepam (Dalmane®). These drugs are used to decrease anxiety, tension, agitation, and insomnia.

Most do not relax muscles directly, but affect brain functioning and feelings. There is no evidence of any direct pain-relieving properties. Although often given for the management of chronic pain, there is little justification for this unless acute anxiety problems are present.

Drowsiness and lethargy are common initial reactions to taking these drugs, but these symptoms gradually decrease as tolerance builds. Physical and psychological dependencies on these drugs may occur, requiring gradual withdrawal. Too rapid a reduction can cause agitation, insomnia, anxiety, nightmares, and tremors.

Antidepressants

Anti-depressants are sometimes prescribed for chronic pain patients. These may be given whether or not the patient has any evidence of clinical depression. Common anti-depressants are amitriptyline (Elavil®), imipramine (Tofranil®), doxepin (Sinequan®), and tranylcypromine (Parnate®). Side-effects that can occur with these drugs, include dry mouth, blurred vision, lethargy, constipation, and sexual dysfunctions.

Muscular Relaxants

Muscular relaxants are often prescribed, and common examples of these are meprobamate (Equanil®), cyclobenzaprine (Flexeril®), methocarbamol (Robaxisal®, Robaxin®). Muscular relaxants vary in their effectiveness from day to day and from patient to patient. Their use should only be on a short-term basis, as there appears to be questionable benefit from chronic use. The possible side-effects are difficulty with concentration, headaches, dizziness, and drowsiness.

Drugs for Specific Pain Complaints

Finally, there are specific drugs that are sometimes prescribed for particular pain problems such as headache. Classical and common migraine are believed to be due to a reduced stability in the inter- and extracranial arteries. This can result in vessel changes, involving overconstriction (at which time the patient may see visual effects). This is followed by a second phase of overdilation of the arteries, in which the patient may feel extreme pain and become nauseous and vomit. The drugs are used in an attempt to reduce these changes, and three types are available. The first are prophylactic drugs, or drugs used daily in order to prevent the onset of headaches. The common drugs of this type are:

1. Methysergide maleate (Sansert®): This drug is one that is used to potentiate the vasoconstriction produced by norepinephrine. Unfortunately, there are a number of side-effects, which include nausea, anxiety, drowsiness, muscular cramps, and weight gain.
2. Propranolol (Inderal®) is used to prevent the vasodilation phase.
3. Clonidine hydrochloride (Catapres®): This is used to reduce both vasoconstriction and vasodilation. The complications of chronic use of this drug are, among other things, depression, retinal degeneration, drowsiness, constipation, and mouth dryness.

Secondly, symptomatic treatment drugs are used to try to control episodes of pain. The most common drugs in this group are:

1. Ergotamine tartrate (Gynergen® and Ergomar®) and ergotamine plus caffeine (Cafergot®). These drugs were produced in order to effect a powerful and prolonged vasoconstriction of the arteries, to counteract the dilation phase of migraine (i.e., to counteract the phase when pain is experienced). These drugs are used at the onset of attacks during the prodromal, or pre-pain, symptoms (visual effects, etc.). Chronic high doses (of ergotamine, etc.) can result in nausea, vomiting, weakness, drowsiness, circulation disturbances, cold skin, muscle pain, angina, tachycardia, changes in blood pressure, and headaches. Fatalities have been reported with excessive doses.
2. A second drug of this sort is pizotyline maleate (Sandomigran®). The side-effects of this drug are weight gain, drowsiness, muscle cramps, restless legs, fluid retention, and dizziness. In some cases, more frequent, milder headaches have been reported, in addition to migraine in some 10% of cases. Some of the additional disturbances are considered due to the adverse effects of antihistamines occurring with pizotyline (headache, blurred vision, nightmares, dizziness, gastrointestinal disturbances, muscle weakness).

Unfortunately, there is little evidence of any long-term effectiveness of ergotamine-type drugs, and with continued and excessive use there is growing evidence that they may cause rather than prevent, headache pain. (Results suggest that there is a type of headache [now called an ergotamine headache] that has identical symptoms to those for which it is prescribed.) In many studies, ergotamine has been shown to be about as effective as a mild analgesic (such as propoxyphene), though unfortunately carrying a number of the disadvantageous side-effects discussed earlier. The worsening of classic and common migraine with drug abuse is now recognized as a potential cause of chronicity of this problem.

Unfortunately, there is a tendency for headache sufferers to start overusing these drugs as they find them decreasingly effective in controlling pain. This gradually leads to an exacerbation or worsening of their whole problem, encouraging further use of more drugs, and have more side-effects. Overall, it is unlikely that this group of drugs is effective over time; in a large survey of headache patients, only 25% felt that any of the drugs they took were effective. For the most part, they continue to use their drugs feeling that if they were not taking the drugs, they would be even worse off.

Sudden withdrawal from any of these drugs should be avoided. Withdrawal must be managed slowly and carefully and should be monitored by an expert to avoid rebound headaches (a resurgence of headache that may occur with the sudden cessation of drugs). Patients trying to rid themselves of the addiction "cold turkey" often find their problems increased, and they quickly return to their drugs with an increased dependence upon them.

Sumitriptan has been shown to effectively abort episodes of migraine (Oral Sumitriptan Study Group, 1991; Rose, 1993; Sheftell & Weeks, 1994) and is well tolerated (Tansey & Pilgrim, 1993; see also Moskowitz & Cutrer, 1993). The longer-term effects of this drug are under investigation.

Conclusion

First, chronic use of analgesics for the control of pain can become increasingly inadequate for relief and often causes physical and psychological dependencies on drugs, as well as unpleasant side-effects that can be more damaging than the original pain. Secondly, it is important for people with chronic pain problems to understand the nature of the drugs they take and the options that are available. Finally, although it is an admirable aim to be entirely drug-free, it may not always be feasible (e.g., degenerative spinal conditions, arthritic problems, cancer pain). However, it is often possible to reduce the analgesic dependence or to shift gradually to a less damaging drug if chronic use is found to be necessary. The aim of treatment is to help patients reach as low a dosage level as possible. As they develop other techniques to manage their pain, the use of drugs can be reduced substantially or even eliminated.

Problem Solving

The effect of this group discussion can make some patients eager to begin withdrawal immediately, or even to stop on the spot! Although this may be the ultimate goal of training, it is unwise to act precipately. Patients have few coping strategies by Session #4 and are likely to overreact to pain episodes experienced once they are off the drug, and quickly resume drug use. Gradual and controlled reduction is by far the best approach. It can be stressed to them at this point that they will be in a much better position to manage without the drug once they have learned the many skills involved in the treatment program. The graduated method of withdrawal gives them a chance to learn these techniques and ensures that the changes they make will be enduring. In addition, it is worth pointing out once again that the withdrawal symptoms from many of the drugs are unpleasant but can be minimized or prevented by a sensibly organized medication reduction program. As the patient's confidence grows in his or her capacity to manage pain, the psychological dependency will also begin to reduce. (The importance of psychological factors is evident from, among other factors, the analgesic power of non-specific, placebo treatments [Turner et al., 1994]). Thus, keep in mind that as well as reducing a physical dependency, the therapist is also guiding the patient in the reduction of a psychological dependency on drug taking. The latter is best extinguished or reduced by gradual methods that give the patient a sense of control over events, as well as time to integrate the new methods or techniques when faced with intense pain episodes.

GRADUATED REDUCTION PROGRAM (TACTIC #3)

Two tactics are focused on during the practical section of this session: drug reduction and relaxation induction (continued). The first and most important topic is a detailed description of how drugs can be withdrawn in a way that minimizes side-effects and how to integrate the skill training provided in the treatment program. The reduction of drugs often provokes some anxiety, even after a decision has been made to reduce and hopefully eliminate the drugs during treatment. Hence, it is essential to describe to patients a structured program that will help them toward their goal.

Regular Timed Medication Schedules

Emphasize the importance of regular medication use on a timed basis rather than medication based on pain increments. Regular intake of medication has a more powerful effect on pain management than the sporadic intake of drugs. The latter is the method that often evolves in the attempt of chronic pain patients not to use drugs unless they feel it is necessary. Although commendable, this tends to lead them to use the drug only when the pain is at such a level that little therapeutic benefit will come from the ingestion of the drug (especially as tolerance increases). In addition, anxiety may arise as pain increments, and lead to an increase in the level of pain experienced.

With chronic pain, a better method of using drugs is to take them at regular intervals. The taking of the drug is determined by the movement of the clock rather than by changes in pain experienced. Connections begin to erode between drug taking and relief from pain, and the patients interrupt their continuous concern about whether or not the moment to take drugs has arrived. It is also possible that anxiety about pain is lower with this type of scheduling, although this has not been experimentally investigated. Pain may be better managed because, with the regular intake of a prescribed drug, the amount of drug within the blood is sustained at a more constant level throughout the day. There is less chance, therefore, that the level of pain will rise out of control.

Regular scheduling is the first step that needs to be taken prior to beginning a reduction program. It is easier to reduce drug intake once patients are on this regular schedule. Patients with patterns of episodic drug use may need reassurance at the outset. They can be asked to take drugs on some occasions when they would have been able to manage without them, and they may be concerned about increasing their use of drugs by doing so. Remind them that the average level of their drug taking has been assessed and that they are being given a proportion of their average daily dose at each of three or four points. They will find that, with this method, the pain becomes less intense and more manageable. If properly organized, they should have no reason to expect or need to increase their drug intake because of the change to a regular time-based program.

The Use of a Liquid Medication Equivalent

Once patients are on a schedule of taking their pills three to four times a day, the gradual reduction of the drug is made easier by shifting them to the use of a liquid equivalent of their usual capsule or pill. Capsules cannot be accurately cut into smaller and smaller pieces, and thus the control of the dosage reduction is inaccurate. In addition, once patients are on a liquid equivalent, the volume of each dose can remain constant by gradually increasing the neutral solution as the drug decreases. In this way, there is no feeling of loss of medication in terms of amount of medication received. The active pharmacological ingredient can be suspended in a neutral solution. It is important at the start of this switch from pills to liquid medication that the patient should have time to adjust to the liquid form of the drug. Some people have difficulty making this transition and may need more than a week to adjust to it. The use of a liquid medication equivalent prescription incidentally capitalizes on the powerful nonspecific analgesic effects of neutral substances that are used in the context of pain-reduction procedures.

This is a rough outline of a reduction program, giving the percentage reductions over a nine-week period:

Week 1: Medication taken 3 to 4 times daily by the clock.
Week 2: Liquid equivalent of the drug 3 to 4 times daily: 100% of the original dose level.
Week 3: Same as above.
Week 4: Similar scheduling; 10% reduction from original dose level to 90% of original.
Week 5: Similar scheduling; 25% reduction from original dose to 75% .

Week 6: Similar scheduling; 45% reduction from original dose to 55% level.

Week 7: Similar scheduling; 65% reduction from original dose to 35% level.

Week 8: Similar scheduling; 85% reduction from original dose to 15% level.

Week 9: Similar scheduling; 100% reduction from original dose to 0% level.

This rough guide can be modified in light of a patient's reaction to it. At this point, it is important for patients to know the standard regime of reduction being used, while being reassured that this reduction program will be modified to meet their particular needs (e.g., some patients will not need a second week on the liquid equivalent and can move straight into the first 10% reduction; another patient may not be comfortable with a further 15% reduction at week 7 and would like to reduce only 10%). This example should be taken as a skeleton reduction program and modified according to the particular needs of the patients involved.

Some patients do not wish to know how they are progressing, and ask the pharmacist to make all the necessary reductions once they have chosen to undertake the program. Others like to see exactly what they have achieved and wish the percentage reduction to be indicated on their bottles of medication. There is no justification for, nor any wisdom in, any deceit between the patient, therapist, and pharmacist. Full disclosure and reinforcement of the patients by the expert on the problem is essential.

Graded Reductions

The timing of reductions is important and should be undertaken in a way that gives patients maximum control. If it is practical and feasible, the best arrangement is for patients to make any changes in their reduction schedule in conjunction with the therapist at a session, picking up their prescriptions immediately afterwards. This allows negotiations to occur. Patients acquire a sense of control and the opportunity to slow up the reduction program should they feel the need to do so. The majority of patients will not need to do this, but giving them the option places control in their own hands and makes them less fearful about the reduction program. On occasions, when patients slow up the reduction, they may have a tendency to feel a failure, especially when the majority of the group is reducing on schedule. This can be dealt with by praising them for taking command of the situation and deciding to slow up the reduction. Again, the individual differences in response to a program can be emphasized and a patient commended for being wise enough to slow up drug reduction while he or she strengthens skills further.

Dealing with Temptation

Patients should be advised at this stage that they may feel a desire to supplement the drugs being given by adding additional drugs (e.g., Frosst 222s), or by supplementing the drug regime with new drugs (decongestants, laxatives). This is to be discouraged, and reported to the therapist or pharmacist on the next session. They can also be advised to throw away any extra unused pills. The temptation of bottles of pills in the cupboard can be explained to patients. If they are concerned about the financial loss involved, the pills can be handed in and retained for the patients until the end of treatment. At that point, patients can make a wiser decision about whether they wish to keep their drugs.

Problem Solving

"Doctor Shopping"

Occasionally, a patient will weaken in his or her resolve to continue the reduction program, and may seek alternative prescriptions elsewhere ("doctor shopping"). Any doctor shopping, it should be made clear, will lead to the patient being asked to leave the program and their treatment terminated. The program requires a cooperative and constructive relationship between therapist and patient, and secrecy and deceit are not acceptable. Patients selecting themselves for this type of self-management approach are very unlikely to fall into these types of patterns, but occasionally a patient may find him or herself inclined to do this, especially if the program appears to be going faster than he or she can manage. Thus, it is important to emphasize the fact that although a set routine has been established, patients can negotiate, at any time, to slow up the reduction process.

Inappropriate Scheduling or Loss of Prescription

From the outset, it is important to take a very firm stance with respect to problems that may arise for patients during the week, when they are at home and managing the problem without the therapist's help. Prescriptions are filled only once a week, before or after the session, by the pharmacist who is working with the psychologist. If bottles are broken or lost, the patients will have to manage on their own devices until the week is up. The pharmacist measures precisely the amount needed for the patient over that period, and it is the patient's responsibility to make this last. If all the medication is used up on the first day, due to irregular medication schedule or excessive medication use, medication will not last. The prescribed sequence will give the best coverage over the whole week. If the patient is able to regain a prescription or acquire supplementary doses, this erodes the determination and leads back to the previous routine, wherein the pain was reinforced by analgesic prescriptions. This firmness needs to be handled in a nonpunitive manner. Discuss the arrangement with the patients at the start, so that they know the conditions under which they do, or do not, get prescriptions. For the majority of patients, this particular discussion is unnecessary. However, for a few, who are extremely dependent or have had problems obtaining medications from their doctors, it is important to be clear on these issues. Needless to say, this method demands that the therapist and pharmacist involved be the *only* prescribers. This must be established with the referring physician from the start of the program.

PROGRESSIVE RELAXATION WITH CALMING/ DISTRACTING IMAGERY (CONTINUATION OF TACTICS #1A AND #1B AND INTRODUCTION OF TACTIC #5)

The second section of this practical period is used to reinforce and teach relaxation methods. In addition, a further dimension touches on the fifth tactic (Distraction), which is introduced at a later stage as one of a number of focusing techniques. However, its introduction at this point is a useful addition to the relaxation skill, strengthening it and providing another method of control.

Relaxation is induced (as in Session #2), watching for any difficulties that patients are having with the relaxation induction or breathing techniques. Following approximately 15 minutes of induction, the last five minutes are spent on the use of imagery (peaceful and antagonistic to pain experience). Specific images are suggested to patients, and toward the end of the 5-minute period they are encouraged to generate their own. It is explained that the use of peaceful imagery in conjunction with their deep relaxation work can act to reduce pain experience. The fact that they have managed to reduce the tension level in their bodies and attain a state of increasing physical relaxation will not necessarily lead to a calm, relaxed mental state. Specific peaceful images are potent in helping to achieve this. Allow a full 5 minutes for their experimentation with different personal images, suggesting that they think of events or settings from the past that are associated with great calm, pieces of music they feel are tranquilizing, and so forth. The therapist may need to provide specific images (e.g., lying in a warm bath, sunbathing on a sandy beach) for some patients who have difficulty with imaginal work. Providing specific images can be difficult in group work because of the variation between people in the images that can induce a tranquilizing influence; it is better undertaken in individual sessions.

Following the work on deep relaxation and emotional imagery, allow time for a general discussion of their increasing capacity to relax and the effect of introducing imagery into this process. A number of factors influence the capacity of a person to concentrate on imagery and to gain a calming effect. Make sure that the distinction between their body being relaxed and their mind being relaxed is understood and that they recognize the importance of attempting an integration of the two. Those with intense pain during the relaxation period need to be encouraged to "ride over the pain" in their attempts to relax despite it. This is a highly concentrated task and will demand encouragement from the therapist. The muscular relaxation work can be extended by concentrated work on mental imagery.

Problem Solving

Patients who experience difficulty in generating images may need verbal reminders to explore color, light, shape, light patterns, sound, and even kinesthetic memories in elaborating their image. They will also need encouragement to explore which particular images will produce a tranquilizing effect. It is wise for patients to generate two or three such images, so that when working daily on their relaxation tapes, they can vary the image. Continually using one image when relaxing can lead to its fading and becoming less potent.

HOMEWORK ASSIGNMENTS

Continuing Assignments

Increase the demand at this stage for daily exercise quotas, tailoring them to each person in light of their response to the previous homework. Those ready to make the first drug reduction will be moving down to 90% of their original dose, while some in the group may be maintained at 100% until they have adjusted to the liquid analgesic.

Encourage the continuing use of relaxation twice daily, with an additional 5 minutes in which they attend to relaxing, calming images in order to extend the relaxation effect still further.

Monitoring Stress Events

In preparation for the next week's focus, ask patients to monitor stressful events that occur during the week. If weekly diaries have been made for patients in which they monitor the pain levels (see Figure 6.2), it may be possible for them to monitor stress levels in the upper portion of their diaries, thus allowing them to note the connections between pain variations (peaks and troughs) and difficult events they have had to deal with during the week. Their notes need not be extensive; they merely act as reminders of an event that has occurred. Often it is only later that the significance of certain events with respect to pain increment/decrement becomes clear. Encourage patients to use their diaries as a way of accumulating evidence on associations (e.g., severe migraine headaches occurring the day after a dinner party).

SUGGESTED READINGS

Aronoff, G. M., Wagner, J. M., & Spangler, A. S. (1986). Chemical interventions for pain. *Journal of Consulting and Clinical Psychology, 54*(6), 769–775.

Foley, K. M. (1985). Adjuvant analgesic drugs in cancer pain management. In G.M. Aronoff (Ed.), *Evaluation and treatment of chronic pain* (pp. 425–434). Baltimore, MD: Urban & Schwarzenberg.

Fordyce, W. E. (1976). *Behavioral methods for chronic pain and illness.* St. Louis, MO: Mosby.

Holroyd, K. A., & Penzien, D. B. (1990). Pharmacological versus non-pharmacological prophylaxis of recurrent migraine headache: A meta-analytic review of clinical trials. *Pain, 42,* 1–13.

Kudrow, L. (1982). Paradoxical effects of frequent analgesic use. In M. Critchley (Ed.), *Advances in neurology: Vol. 33,* (pp. 335–343). New York: Raven Press.

Moskowitz, M. A., & Cutrer, F. M. (1993). Sumatriptan: A receptor targeted treatment for migraine. *Annual Review of Medicine, 44,* 145–154.

Oral Sumitriptan International Multiple-Dose Study Group. (1991). Evaluation of a multiple-dose regimen of oral sumatriptan for the acute treatment of migraine. 8th Migraine Trust International Symposium: Sumatriptan: From molecule to man. In *European Neurology, 31,* 316–333.

Rose, F. C. (1993). Sumatriptan: An overview. *Headache Quarterly, 4,* 37–41.

Sarkis, E., & Turner, J. A. (1982). Self-report versus actual use of medication in chronic pain patients. *Pain, 12,* 285–294.

Turner, J. A., & Calsyn, D. A. (1982). Drug utilization patterns in chronic pain patients. *Pain, 12,* 357–363.

Turner, J. A., Deyo, R. A., Loeser, J. D., Von Korff, M., & Fordyce, W. E. (1994). The importance of placebo effects in pain treatment and research. *Journal of the American Medical Association, 271,* 1609–1614.

White, B., & Saunders, S. H. (1985). Differential effects on pain and mood in chronic pain with time versus pain contingent medication delivery. *Behavior Therapy, 60*(1), 28–39.

CHAPTER 11

The Role of Emotional State (Session #5)

REVIEW OF PREVIOUS ASSIGNMENTS

At this fifth week of treatment, there is little need to spend much time in reviewing the exercise program, relaxation work, or drug reduction program. Patients will feel accustomed to the graded nature of the program and may merely need a quick reminder and further encouragement to continue on their own.

At this stage, the treatment plan is halfway to completion, and it is also useful to remind the patients of the progress they have made to date. They will have made the initial steps in improving their fitness and activity levels, in learning to manage muscular tension and breaking the links between tension and chronic pain, and in reducing, at least a little, their dependence on drugs. From this basis, it is possible to move on to more precise control techniques, which are emphasized from this session onward. Patients will need to continue working on each of the tactics previously introduced but will complement them with the more finely tuned cognitive behavioral tactics. Emphasize the major step that they have already made toward fulfilling many of the goals that they had set for themselves. They may wish to look once again at their goal sheets after the session to check on this. However, most of this review section of the session can best be spent in encouraging members of the group to describe the conclusions they have drawn from their pain diaries and monitoring over the last week. Any patterns that they have noted in relation to events, emotional periods, frustrations and difficulties, and so forth, will be useful illustrations of the interrelationship between emotional reactions and pain levels, which is the focus of Session #5.

THE ROLE OF EMOTIONAL STATE

The Relationship of Emotions and Chronic Pain

For a number of sessions, the therapist has concentrated attention on the vicious cycle that can develop between muscular tension and chronic pain. The tactics taught have been designed to help the patient break the cycle that develops in response to continuing pain, and thus to reduce pain levels.

At about this stage in treatment, having done considerable self-monitoring of pain levels, patients are in a position to turn their attention to the vicious cycle that can develop between their chronic pain problem and their emotional state. In discussing this subject when treatment is well underway, and by having had time to monitor their own emotional reactions in relation to pain experienced, they will approach this subject with less apprehension.

The aim of the session is to introduce the subject of the interplay between emotions and pain, explaining how patients may inadvertently contribute to their own pain problems by their emotional reactions. Understanding this influence on pain levels will inspire patients to work toward reducing and, one hopes, breaking the vicious cycle that may be operating.

Severe episodes of pain and the continuing and ever-present disruption of life they cause, lead to increasing anxiety in the face of each episode or each increment in pain experienced. It is not surprising that, as pain mounts, the person feels a sense of impotence in managing it and a fear about how he or she will deal with such episodes in the future. As with any other upsetting or aversive event, the sufferer will notice that his or her muscle tension increases. In addition, the heart may race, the legs feel weak, the palms feel sweaty, and patients may feel fatigued and preoccupied with their condition. Some people feel themselves to be increasingly moody and often become entangled with the experience of pain itself. Over time, it becomes increasingly difficult to differentiate the experience of anxiety from the feelings of pain. Thus, the emotional reaction to pain or to other provoking stimuli may become part of the experience of pain itself.

Unfortunately, emotional reactions to pain can contribute to a person's intolerance for pain. The more tense and agitated the person becomes, the worse the pain episode will become and the longer it will last. This is the core of the vicious cycle that is illustrated in Figure 7.3 and is the focus of the session.

Unfortunately it is not only the reactions to pain that contribute to the emotional state of the chronic pain sufferer. Other situations and difficulties can contribute to the emotional turmoil a person may feel (anxiety, tension, anger). These in turn will begin to affect pain tolerance. Needless to say, the types of situations that produce increments in emotionality will vary between patients. The anxiety of bringing up children and the responsibilities that this entails may be potent for one; for another, work pressures and self-imposed high standards may prove stressful. For one person, relationships may be the focus of his or her emotional reactions, while for another it may be his or her isolation and loneliness that provokes distress.

Pain can be elevated by anxiety, tension, or anger. The best explanation for the incrementations of pain by these emotions is contained in the Gate Control Model, explained in the first session. Heightened emotionality is one of the factors that ''opens the gate'' and can produce the central disinhibition of afferent impulses. Thus, under conditions of high arousal and emotionality, it is likely that the person will feel more pain, irrespective of the reason for this increment in emotion. However, there is some suggestion that where the anxiety is focused upon pain, the detrimental effects on tolerance are greater (Weisenberg, Aviram, Wolf, & Rafael, 1984).

Emphasis should be given to the fact that although emotional reactions are not *the cause* of pain, they undoubtedly make a great difference in the capacity of the person to manage his or her own pain problem. Anxiety and anger produce many similar physical effects on a person, and the above remarks are equally applicable to high levels of frustration and anger. The overlap of physical sensation produced by severe pain, high levels of anxiety, or anger and frustration is worth emphasizing. When the reactions are comparable under different conditions, it is easy to confuse the emotional state with the pain problem. Muscles become tight, the heart races, breathing becomes faster, and sweating occurs under all three conditions. Encourage members of the group to give examples of occasions during the last week in which they noticed these physical changes in themselves, either with or without pain increments. It is also useful to encourage a discussion of the confusion between emotional and physical pains.

Dampening or Defusing Emotional Reactions

In the latter part of the didactic section, encourage a more practical and focused approach to how such reactions can be reduced in order to minimize pain, and increase pain tolerance. Emotional reactions can be heightened or dampened under certain conditions. When they are dampened, the impact of events is reduced. Encourage members of the group to illustrate this idea from their own experience (e.g., "When I am having a bad pain episode, I get very upset by loud noises made by the children, and my pain feels much worse.") Some people are much better than others at delineating the events or situations that enlarge emotions and those, in contrast, that can dampen or reduce them. The self-monitoring done the week prior is a useful and practical first step and can be drawn on by the therapist at this stage of the session. Individual differences in provoking stimuli, and the effect of these stimuli on pain peaking, can be pointed out.

In addition, patients may be able to delineate the very small adjustments in themselves that herald the beginning of anxiety or anger. Encourage patients to focus on the physical changes in their muscles and bodies so that they can become increasingly sensitive to the adjustments of their own bodies in the face of stress. Physical tension usually builds up gradually; it can be associated with slight changes in breathing, gastric sensations in the pit of the stomach, damp palms, and a feeling of unease. Since there are large differences between people in the ways in which they manifest emotions, each person needs to evaluate his or her own reaction pattern in order to become more sensitive to the small but early signs of emotion. Detecting these changes is a useful addition to the self-monitoring of pain and starts a process of differentiating emotional reactions from pain episodes. In addition, it is important for patients to become aware of the small physical changes that herald emotional reactions in order to utilize the defusing strategy to be introduced in the practical section of this session.

In addition to detecting small physical changes, it is important to consider ways in which patients may be able to pace their own activities and involvement so as to maintain a sense of calm and control and to minimize build-ups of emotionality during the day. Establishing regular times to do relaxation training, using calming imagery in order to dampen an emotional build-up, is worth their consideration. Breaks in their activity and "time off" from frustrations can be programmed into their day (e.g., a busy switchboard operator may have to be persuaded to take regular breaks and or two-minute periods in which no calls are dealt with and deep diaphragmatic breathing is undertaken).

Such steps become active ways of reducing anxiety or the build-up of anger. When anger or anxiety is provoked by pain episodes themselves, relaxation can be a potent method for counteracting the build-up. It is important to encourage the use of this technique early on in the evolution of a pain episode rather than leaving it until the pain is unmanageable. Further methods will be taught as treatment progresses, but at this stage, emphasize the importance of utilizing the early signs of agitation as cues to introduce relaxation methods. It is likely that the earlier these techniques are used, the stronger their effect.

DEFUSING EMOTIONAL REACTIONS (TACTIC #4)

During this practical section of the session, it is useful to demonstrate the defusing technique that patients can practice in the face of stress reactions.

Induce relaxation over a 15-minute period, asking the patients to concentrate, toward the end, on a peaceful, calming image. Once satisfied that they are relaxing and breathing regularly in a deep fashion, ask them to switch to a stimulus that has, in the past, provoked anxiety or anger. For those unable to generate such a stimulus, ask them to use their memory of the last severe episode of pain they endured. Call their attention to the physical changes they note in their own bodies as their minds move from the peaceful images over to the anxiety of anger-provoking images. Give them enough time to notice changes, and then give instructions to breathe evenly and steadily, asking them to maintain the image while they relax completely. If relaxation training has been proceeding well and has been practiced fully between sessions, the idea of the out breath as a relaxation cue can be suggested at this point and associated with the diminution of anxiety as relaxation is superimposed.

After they begin to notice the physical changes associated with the anxiety-provoking stimulus, they are encouraged to breathe them away, using the out breath and increasing their relaxation further. An example of this type of defusing technique is as follows: The patients are well relaxed, breathing evenly and steadily, thinking about a peaceful scene. Ask them to imagine the way they felt on the last occasion they had to deal with a difficult relation, and on the first detection of physical changes in themselves to breathe out, breathing away the tension and relaxing further and further as they continue to think of the occasion.

The above demonstration draws upon a well-established behavioral technique, namely, systematic desensitization (Wolpe, 1958). Behavior therapists will be acquainted with this type of methodology for the management of anxiety stimuli. (Those with no experience of such techniques are advised to read the suggested reference list before proceeding.) The importance of the practical demonstration of the potency of relaxation techniques is that it gives patients a sense of their own power to control their stress reactions. When anxiety induced by this stimulus also produces changes in pain experienced, the patient's use of relaxation methods will illustrate to him or her the potency of this strategy in reducing pain. It will illustrate:

1. the link between emotional state and pain levels;
2. the relationship between anxiety reduction and pain levels; and
3. the fact that the person can utilize a control tactic to counteract the negative consequences of these interrelationships.

Encourage patients in the group to delineate the physical changes they felt while thinking of the emotionally provoking stimulus. To what extent did it affect their pain experience or the muscle groups associated with their pain focus? For example, a patient with facial pain spontaneously reported after this exercise a massive increase in muscular tightening and tension of her jaw when she thought about an anxiety-provoking scene. This resulted in an increase of facial pain. Defusing anxiety in the way described above led to the pain gradually subsiding.

Summarize toward the end of this practical section the suggested steps for the defusing and dampening of emotional reactions and the control of pain. In the first place, it is necessary that each person clarify for him or herself the events, situations, and emotions that are provoking increases in pain or agitation. Patterns often emerge while self-monitoring is on-going.

The second step is to try to identify the small, detectable physical changes that herald the onset of an emotional reaction to pain or other situations and stimuli. Early perception is to be encouraged, as well as identification or specific early cues that may be idiosyncratic. Third, relaxation techniques can be used to dampen pain and overreactivity and are especially forceful if used at the onset of an emotional reaction. In addition to specific relaxation techniques, patients should consider the feasibility of pacing activities, both at home and at work, so that a sense of calm and control can be maintained and a build-up of tension minimized.

Problem Solving

The Use of Imagery

There is considerable variability in the capacity of people to imagine anxiety-provoking situations. Sometimes concentration is affected by being part of a group. In addition, some people are poor at evoking visual memories and may need to be encouraged to generate thoughts or memories from the past that provoke emotional reactions. Imagining a recent severe pain episode may be more potent for some people than for others. In a group setting, the therapist depends on each person to generate a provocative imaginal stimulus; and you expect that the potency will vary between patients, depending on how effectively they are able to undertake this task.

The Necessity of Practice

An initial demonstration can sometimes produce powerful effects on people; however, many patients may need to try on a number of occasions before the linkages between emotion and pain are clearly demonstrated or their capacities to defuse these reactions are clarified. As with all other skill learning, the more practice they have with the techniques, the more adept they will become in using them. Starting with imaginal stimuli makes the task somewhat easier in that the imaginal stimulus will seldom produce an excessive amount of emotion to be defused.

Denials

Some people will forcefully deny that they ever feel anxious or upset or that they ever have reason to be angry. These people will be greatly aided by hearing the discussion of the group, in which there are always some members who are aware of and discuss the important linkages they have noticed between their emotional reactions and their pain problems. Continuing their monitoring can be a useful task for such people by placing the emphasis on the monitoring of emotional reactions independent of their relationship to pain. In the meantime, ask them to deal with their reactions to excessive pain, seeing if they can defuse and reduce them by the relaxation method. Their focus can be entirely upon such physical cues as the fast breathing or racing heart that often accompanies severe pain episodes.

HOMEWORK ASSIGNMENTS

Practice of the New Tactics

The important addition to their array of techniques to be practiced between sessions is the use of defusing techniques in the face of an intense pain or of anxiety. They may find it useful to indicate on their self-monitoring diaries when stress events occurred and the degree of success they had in counteracting them. Those unsure about the early sensations at the onset of a bout of extreme anxiety or anger can be encouraged to indicate these early cues on their self-monitoring sheets as well.

Exercise quotas can be increased again this week in conjunction with the decreasing drug levels (using the graded reduction method).

Preparation for the Next Session

The role of attention focus is the next topic to be considered. In preparation for this, a helpful homework assignment for patients is to monitor the amount of time they talk about their pain or disability during the week. It is often useful for a spouse or partner to also undertake this task independently of the patient. Monitoring forms can be provided for them, and an example of the type of sheet that can be utilized is shown in Appendix IX. The discrepancies between patient and spouse or partner are of great interest on some occasions, but it is often hard to enlist the participation of a relative in this task. The reason for this may prove important (lack of interest, irritation, lack of empathy) and may be a relevant consequence of the continuing pain problem, which will be useful for each patient to understand. These issues are raised in the next session but are of considerably more impact if the patient has been asked to undertake a certain amount of self-monitoring prior to the discussion.

SUGGESTED READINGS

Eich, E., Rachman, S., & Lopatka, C. (1990). Affect, pain, and autobiographical memory. *Journal of Abnormal Psychology, 99,* 174–178.

Graceley, R. H., McGraff, P., & Dubner, R. (1978). Validity and sensitivity of ratio scales or sensory and effective verbal pain descriptors: Manipulation of effect by diazepam. *Pain, 5,* 19–29.

Melzack, R., & Wall, P. (1988). *The challenge of pain.* Harmondsworth, Middlesex, England: Penguin Books.

Weisenberg, M., Aviram, D., Wolf, Y., & Raphael, I. N. (1984). Relevant and irrelevant anxiety in the reaction to pain. *Pain, 20*(4), 371–385.

Wolpe, J. (1958). *Psychotherapy by reciprocal inhibition.* Stanford, Stanford University Press.

CHAPTER 12

The Role of Attention Focus and Complaint (Session #6)

REVIEW OF PREVIOUS ASSIGNMENTS

By this stage in treatment, members of the group will automatically begin by giving their reactions to their homework tasks. The therapist reinforces and encourages any suggestion of increasing exercise and application of relaxation routines, as well as persistence with drug reduction. Try to refrain from asking about their pain during the previous week, focusing attention on what they have been able to achieve despite their pain. The fact that exercise has been increasing, while drugs have been reduced, can be emphasized at this stage, and a diagram of the crossover effect can be drawn on a blackboard to illustrate their progress.

Discussion of Pain and Disability

Most of the preliminary period is best spent upon a discussion of the monitoring of expressions of pain distress and complaint. The group members can be encouraged to look for discrepancies between their own view of the problem and that of their spouses or friends (as long as it was done without the patient's help). As mentioned, difficulties may arise in obtaining a partner's participation in this task. Some partners will undermine the investigation by the patient or refuse to undertake it themselves. It is useful to encourage a discussion of why this might have occurred, as it illustrates the material to be discussed in the didactic portion (regarding response of others to chronic pain complaint). Group discussion is often helpful to patients in their attempts to understand the implications of a spouse's refusal to monitor (e.g., lack of interest, adaptation/satisfaction, hostility, anxiety regarding the effects of the treatment program on the patient's behavior).

THE ROLE OF ATTENTION FOCUS AND COMPLAINT

Somatic Focusing

A common consequence of a chronic pain problem is the tendency to focus increasingly on pain sensation itself: its qualities, its extent, and its spread. In addition, sufferers can find themselves preoccupied with the limitations that pain imposes on their lives. Other interests may be neglected, and attention may become focused almost exclusively on the internal state of their bodies (e.g., the way the face feels, the way the head aches, the way the back pulls). In talking to others, they may find themselves constantly bringing up the issue that is foremost in their minds. It may not always be in terms of the intensity of the pain they are suffering but may take the form of a discussion of medicines, appointments with doctors, encroaching disability, and catastrophic predictions about ultimately becoming an invalid. The didactic presentation in this session deals with the role of attention focus upon pain and the indirect effect this focusing can have upon relationships with others. Complaint of pain is viewed as *one* type of focusing on pain, which, like other focusing strategies, tends to *decrease* pain tolerance or increase the awareness of pain. Talking and complaining of pain may become an indirect way of controlling others and fulfilling needs. Seen in this way, complaining to friends and relations may be an unassertive method of achieving other goals (i.e., gaining help with the washing up, reducing the number of chores, limiting the demands of children and spouse). Thus, the subject of attention focus is one that leads the therapist to discuss (1) the effects of focus on pain level; (2) the effect of focus on conversation with others; and (3) the effect of pain focus and complaining on the fulfillment of a person's needs. Approaching the subject of "secondary gain" or manipulative behavior in this manner keeps the level of discussion very much in line with the orientation given in the first session. It considers how shifting the focus away from pain may affect the "gate," and how increasing direct expression of needs may break through habitual patterns that have become counterproductive.

This session can be demanding for the therapist if all three areas need to be extensively undertaken with the group. Often the assertion issue need only be touched on as an approach to considering the inappropriateness of manipulating others via pain complaint. People with major problems in asserting themselves may be unsuitable candidates for a group setting and best treated on their own, when a number of sessions can be spent in helping them to resolve the difficulty.

A key aim for the therapist to keep in mind for this session is to provide patients with an understanding of the effect of their attention focus on pain levels. The normality of such a shift of attention should be highlighted first. Chronic pain patients invariably develop a habit of focusing on the sensations in their body, which is understandable and quite adaptive with acute injury. As time passes, however, this overattention to bodily sensations becomes counterproductive with respect to pain management and to their relationships with others.

The Effect of Attention on Pain Levels

Attention can be likened to a spotlight that accentuates the object on which it is focused. By contrast, all other objects outside the circle of the light are in shadows or in darkness and will appear unclear, distant, and less relevant. When the spotlight is on pain sensation and experience, it will highlight this experience and appear to enlarge it. Remembering the Gate Control framework, patients will recognize that attention focus is one of the central influences that widens the gate, preventing any inhibition of messages rising to the brain. By far the best example of this phenomenon is the excruciating pain that can be felt by a person struggling to sleep at night in a dark, unstimulated context of his or her bedroom. The focus of attention is entirely upon the pain, and under such conditions, pain tolerance plummets. In contrast, turning on the lights, listening to a TV program, being entertained by a humorous friend, going downstairs and cooking a midnight feast are activities that can distract and divert the person's attention away from the pain. They have a potent effect of diminishing the pain sensation by partially closing the ''gate.''

The Effect of Attention on Relationships

As time passes and pain persists or increases, it is not surprising that pain is constantly on the sufferer's mind. Gradually, the content of his or her discussions with other people will change and become filled with reference to the pain and its consequences. Various types of disruption of personal relationships follow from this. Initially, it may produce a considerable increase in attention from others and a demonstration of their concern to help in many different ways. In the short-term, there may be comfort from the discussion with others and useful advice offered. Unfortunately, as the pain persists, others may become bored and withdraw from the sufferer. Sometimes this leads to even more vigorous demands for help and attention, with increasing levels of discussion of pain and demonstrations of the difficulties. At this stage, the sufferer's behavior (talking, gestures, and overt behavior) may become an indirect way of seeking the kinds of attention and sustenance that they feel is being withheld, or that has been restricted by their own level of activity and withdrawal. Many chronic pain patients report that a distance begins to grow between them and others, and they feel that the closeness of their relationships has somehow been damaged by their disability. Unable to participate in many of the activities that had been rewarding, they find that contact with others becomes one of the only sources of emotional comfort. Sometimes when people describe their pain, they may be attempting to obtain some sort of sympathy and understanding rather than to directly communicate about any aspect of their problems. In fact, the latter may be redundant and slowly decrease in variability. Over many years, a habit develops of talking indirectly about needs and wishes, and using remarks about pain and disability as a way of obtaining fulfillment. These changes are subtle and slow, as in the development of any habit.

Unfortunately, this habit has a paradoxical effect on relationships: gradually it can prevent a person's attainment of the closeness and warmth that he or she seeks. Thus, the short-term effects of talking about pain may produce a demonstration of affection and encouragement, but the long-term effects may be a growing distancing from others and an unassertiveness with regard to the patient's needs.

In addition, talking about pain and demonstrating pain can become excuses for withdrawing from certain tasks that the person finds distasteful, especially when simultaneously dealing with pain. An irritant (unpleasant work conditions, excessive household duties) can be better limited by the indirect discussion of pain than by a direct confrontation of the irritant. For example, a pain problem may become a legitimate excuse in the minds of other people, as well as the sufferer, for *not* undertaking tasks that he or she has never wished to undertake (e.g., driving the car, earning a living).

This subject needs to be discussed with sensitivity. It is easy for pain patients to adopt a defensive position and to justify their current behavior against allegations of "secondary gain." Once in this position, it is difficult for them to cooperate with the therapist in perceiving the counterproductiveness of a particular pattern of behavior or of learning to adjust that pattern to a more favorable one. Emphasize the normality of preoccupations with sensations and the manipulations of others when a person is faced with continuing distress, as well as the normality of others' tendency to withdraw. Avoid discussions of "secondary gain," at least at this stage, and approach this problem in terms of the use of pain talk as an indirect way of controlling events. Encourage the patients to think about what it must be like for their partners or friends to live with them while they are in pain, drawing on their self-monitoring to illustrate the extent to which a discussion rotates around their problems. Living with someone of whom you are fond, but whose pain you cannot rectify, is extremely frustrating and is dealt with in different ways (refusal to listen to discussion, overconcern and reinforcement, anger). The responses of the spouses or partners to the self-monitoring task often gives some clues as to their reactions to the pain problem per se, which may be useful at this point in the discussion.

FOCUSING TECHNIQUES (TACTICS #5 AND #6)

Having identified the tendency to focus attention upon pain and its deleterious effect on pain management, the therapist should spend this section of the session in suggesting ways in which the "spotlight" can be shifted away from pain, and the pain levels themselves diminished. Two tactics are introduced. The first is a cognitive technique (Tactic #5) for shifting the focus from pain to events external to the person. The second (Tactic #6) entails encouraging the patients to start speaking more directly about what they need and minimizing their use of pain or complaints of disability to achieve other ends.

External Focusing: Tactic #5

During this practical section, the therapist can demonstrate to the patients the implications of what he or she has been delineating: in this case, the effect of attention focus on pain levels. After relaxing the patients in a brief 15-minute induction, ask them to focus on their peaceful imagery and undertake a number of deep, slow, diaphragmatic breaths. Once this pattern has been established, ask them to shift their focus entirely onto their pain problem. (If some patients are enjoying a pain-free period during the session, ask them to focus their attention on any physical discomfort or feeling of pressure they are feeling in their body, e.g., where their thighs reach the edge of the chair.) Keep the focus of their attention entirely on the pain or pressure sensations for a 30-second period, encouraging them to notice the scope, intensity, form, and spread of the pain experience.

Immediately following this, ask them to shift their attention to their environment during the next 30 seconds and to count how many different sounds they can detect, and from what distance they can hear them.

Following this, arouse them for a discussion of these two comparative focusing tasks. Highlight the effect of attention, emphasizing the fact that pain levels were much higher during the period in which they focused exclusively on the sensation of pain, while outside noises were probably not detected at all. In comparison, at times when the outside stimuli were being monitored, pain levels dropped or may have been hardly noticeable when they detected the noises in their environment. The noises will have seemed louder and more dominating. This quickly and efficiently demonstrates the power of the focus of attention. In addition, it suggests how patients are able to use attention-focusing methods to modulate pain experience. Talking about, thinking about, complaining about, ruminating about, and worrying about pain all act to focus attention on sensation. On the other hand, activity, involvement, and focusing on stimulation *outside* the body help minimize the pain and close the "gate."

To avoid frustration, patients should be reminded that these techniques are hard to master and entail a good deal of concentration. It will develop with practice. Initially, while the technique is being mastered, it is wise to practice refocusing techniques, using attention on environmental stimuli (sounds, sights, images, colors, memories) when experiencing low levels of pain. It has the effect of lowering pain levels for a period of time, thus acting as a potent *episodic control* management technique. To have expectations that it will lead to immediate and complete cessation of pain only brings frustration and reduced willingness to utilize this technique in the appropriate way. When patients are battling a continuous problem, it is important that they know how to gain periods of time when pain levels subside. A short period of reduced pain experience can act as a great relief, often improving tolerance for a longer period of time.

Problem Solving

A small percentage of patients find that focusing on the pain *reduces* it rather than increases it. When this occurs, draw out the individual differences in reaction to this focusing technique for the group and offer an explanation of why this might be (e.g., that the person has overextended the scope of pain through the years of suffering). The pain begins to feel as if it covers a much wider area than it really does. Being asked to focus *in* and specify the particular spot leads to a shrinking of the problem. (They have come upon another cognitive technique that will be discussed in more detail in the next session.) The importance of individual differences is a major point to make at this stage; it emphasizes the importance and the relevance of each patient trying out a tactic to see if, and how, it suits him or her.

Assertion: Tactic #6

Shifting the "spotlight" from a focus upon pain to stimuli outside themselves can be greatly aided by a number of simple changes. Patients may report continuous inquiries by friends and relatives about their pain problems, which, they will recognize (after the above discussion), are continually bringing their attention back to their pain and therefore "opening the gate." Because of the length of time over which the patients have been suffering their problems, their friends and relatives begin to expect that it would be only polite to begin all conversations and interactions by inquiring about the pain. Conversations may tend to begin, for example, "And how's your back today?" Other people will suggest activities cautiously, asking whether the patient can manage it. Friends begin to feel that unless they make these kinds of inquiries, they will appear to be unsympathetic and uninterested. The patients themselves may begin to feel that the only thing that is worth having is sympathy and concern from others. They may feel neglected when inquiries are omitted. When this point is reached, it is clear that the problem has become central in the person's life.

It is important that the patients be advised to speak with their friends and relatives about how they can best be of help. They can do this much more efficiently by distracting the patients and encouraging them to shift their focus away from pain, to stimuli outside themselves. The patients need to request friends and spouses to ignore any complaint or demonstration of pain and to immediately switch the conversation to other topics. All inquiries should be made with respect to how well the person is getting on, what activities he or she has been undertaking, and the speed of his or her return to normal. When others fail to do this, the patient should be advised to change the subject on his or her own, as quickly as possible, reminding others that they would help most by taking the more positive approach described above.

Remind the patients that at this stage discussion of pain is a habit that will take a few weeks to break. However, cooperation from spouses and friends will make this trend much easier. In addition, they could ask their friends to praise, encourage, and reward any attempts that the patient undertakes to increase their activity and to move toward a more normal pattern of living. Many spouses and friends are glad to be given specific advice on how to help. For many years, they have watched a struggle and been unable to help. Now the patient can tell them exactly how they can help most, in a specific and structured way.

After so many years of using pain as a method of communicating distress and desires, patients must be encouraged to develop more direct ways of achieving these ends. The difference between assertion and aggression is worth discussing with people who feel some confusion about the limits of direct speaking. The therapist's aim is to encourage the patient to replace discussions of pain wherever possible with more direct, firm statements of their needs. Often, if they are able to delineate under what situations they tend to feel unable to speak firmly and directly, it is useful to encourage them to practice this with the group. At this point in treatment, it will be clear to the therapist where the major focus of their unassertiveness lies (i.e., inability to get time alone to work with the relaxation tapes or to exercise, frustration in dealing with their relations). The treatment approach encourages them to make changes week by week in their usual pattern of activity and to develop various skills. Often it is evident that certain patients are having difficulty undertaking the program because of the reaction of others to the changes they wish to make. Examples of these can be brought to the attention of the people involved, and they can be encouraged to practice a much more assertive or direct statement of their needs. Where time allows, some practice in asserting their needs may well be useful, using a role-playing method with each other and with the therapist.

For example, the scenario may be given to the patients in which they have been asked to go by car to visit a relative they dislike. Their responses might have been to discuss the difficulties of car travel given their pain problem or the level of pain they are currently feeling. In examining this in more detail, it may be discovered that they dislike this relative and don't wish to go or that they do not like being driven by their spouse. They are asked to generate alternative, more direct responses to the spouse in order to express their needs without discussion of pain.

It is useful to encourage patients who are having difficulty with these ideas and/or who are evidently having problems being assertive to do some extra reading, such as the book by Alberti and Emmons, *Your Perfect Right* (1982). This book, like many similar ones, encourages patients to define their own rights without doing so at the expense of others.

HOMEWORK ASSIGNMENTS

Communication

The major step to be taken by patients during this week is to discuss the issue of communication with their spouses, partners, or near relatives. They are to request an uninterested response to any complaint or demonstration of pain they may make during the week. In addition, they are to request an interested and reinforcing reaction to any activity or change toward well behavior that they may make. Those with a tendency to be unassertive are to try, even in a small way, to be firmer and more precise in the expression of their own needs, refraining from using pain talk or pain behavior as a way of fulfilling them. If there are only a few patients with such problems in the group, they might specify the situations in which they intend to be more assertive and direct in the next week (e.g., making clear to the boss that they are not going to do more than a legitimate amount of work in an afternoon, requesting a lunch hour rather than rushing to complete a job while nibbling at a sandwich, etc.).

Problem Solving

Defining Assertion Assignments

When there are major assertion problems for any patients in the group, the therapist will have to be skilled in drawing out a suitable low-intensity item for them to begin with in reasserting themselves with their family. The request to discuss the issue of responses to their complaining is itself quite a skilled act, and to undertake it, as a consequence of this session, is a good first step. Remember to assign other assertion tasks in later sessions to strengthen their capacity to speak more directly about their needs and feelings.

The Role of Attention Focus and Complaint (Session #6)

Refraining from Further Self-Monitoring

A negative requirement is now introduced, which is consistent with the didactic discussion. Patients are asked to refrain from using any more pain diaries or monitoring pain levels in any way at all. Such an activity focuses attention on pain levels. This is usually met with a good deal of delight, as patients find the job of filling in pain diaries increasingly boring. Just as they find it boring to keep monitoring their pain levels, so do others find it boring to keep hearing about them; when appropriate, this uncomfortable fact can be introduced into the discussion of homework.

Preparation for Session #7

The next session will focus upon the thoughts that occur almost spontaneously at the onset of a pain episode or when pain becomes increasingly severe. Patients are asked to monitor these thoughts during the next week in order to bring examples of the kind of spontaneous pain evaluations that occur in association with pain. This monitoring prepares the group for a discussion of the role of cognitions in the management of chronic pain.

Continuing Practice

Remind the patients to continue increasing their exercise quotas toward their goal and to utilize their relaxation at any time during the day that they need it, rather than restricting it to practice times. At this stage, they probably are able to generate a relaxation response without the tape and can experiment with how quickly they can produce deep relaxation within the context of their daily life (relaxing the shoulders while driving the car, breathing deeply while talking on the telephone, etc.). Drug reduction continues to occur. If there have been no reasons to slow up the standard program, patients will now be at 50% of their original dose levels.

SUGGESTED READINGS

Alberti, R., & Emmons, M. L. (1982). *Your Perfect Right.* San Luis Obispo, CA: Impact Publishing.

Fordyce, W. E. (1974). Treating chronic pain by contingency management. In J. Bonica (Ed.), *International symposium on pain—Advances in neurology: Vol. 4.* (pp. 583–589). New York: Raven Press.

Fordyce, W. E. (1976). *Behavioral methods for chronic pain and illness.* St. Louis: Mosby.

Holroyd, K. A., Andrasik, E., & Wesbrook, T. (1977). Cognitive control of tension headache. *Cognitive Therapy Research, 1,* 121–133.

McCaul, K. D., & Mallot, J. M. (1984). Distraction and coping with pain. *Psychological Bulletin, 95*(3), 516–533.

Tan, S. Y. (1982). Cognitive and cognitive behavioural methods for pain control: A selective review, *Pain, 12,* 201–228.

Turk, D. C., & Genest, M. (1979). Regulation of pain: The application of cognitive and behavioral techniques for prevention and remediation. In P. Kendall & S. Hollon (Eds.), *Cognitive behavioral interventions: Theory, research and procedures* (pp. 287–318). New York: Academic Press.

CHAPTER 13

The Role of Appraisal of Pain and the Influence of Depression (Session #7)

REVIEW OF PREVIOUS ASSIGNMENTS

Focus of Attention

In the previous session new assignments were given to the group arising out of the discussion of the extent to which the direction of attention could augment pain. Begin this session by encouraging the discussion of the success of each member of the group in reducing his or her discussion of pain with relatives or spouse, and the attempts to turn the focus of attention toward improvements. Where problems were encountered, encourage other members of the group to help find solutions.

Direct Statement of Needs or Feelings

Where assertive tasks were suggested for specific patients in the previous session, follow this up with an inquiry concerning the effects. Clarify what difficulties, if any, they had in refraining from using discussions of pain to control events. Close relatives or partners may have reacted adversely to a growing firmness shown by the patient. It is often wise to draw patients' attention to the adjustments that will be necessary for their relatives as they begin to move away from their invalid roles. Depending on the success of attempts to be more assertive, further assignments can be set for the next week.

Monitoring Reactions to Pain Episodes

The preparation for the current sessions led patients to monitor their reactions to pain episodes or increases in pain level. Encourage each member of the group to offer one or two samples of his or her "self-talk" in order to demonstrate the types of reactions that are common among persons suffering chronic pain.

THE ROLE OF PAIN APPRAISAL AND DEPRESSION

Cognitive Reactions to Chronic Pain

Persisting and often intense pain problems are preoccupying. The experience is continuously and repeatedly being evaluated or appraised in various ways. Although people vary with respect to the precise form of the thoughts that occur to them, there is considerable similarity in the type of appraisals that are made. Commonly, patients report a feeling of puzzlement and frustration: "Why me?" "Why do I always have the pain?" Sometimes they begin to wonder how they will manage in the future, formulating a thought such as "I am going crazy with this pain. I'm not going to be able to manage my life in the future." They will become concerned with what they *can't* do. If they can't even manage their pain, they may evaluate themselves as "hopeless" or "useless." Ruminating about how long the pain will go on (days, weeks, forever), they may come to the conclusion that they will *never* be free of the pain. If never free of the pain, they may conclude that they will end up doing nothing at all with their lives and that their future will be a total disaster. Often at the onset of a severe pain episode, they may think to themselves, "Well today is a write-off, so there's no point in trying to do anything." Or similarly, "It hurts when I exercise so I can't and I won't move more than I must."

In clarifying the cognitive reactions to pain, the therapist should use, whenever possible, examples reported by the patients from their self-monitoring (see previous examples). Illustrate in the discussion of pain appraisal that often the reactions of chronic pain patients are overreactions to a specific situation, in which they overestimate their disability and predict catastrophe (e.g., "I can't do this task now . . . therefore my life is a total disaster"). The effect of this appraisal is to enlarge the difficulty or the distress and to focus the attention again on the problem. In addition, the evaluations that are made are predominantly, if not exclusively, *negative*. They are negative with respect to the person's capacity to manage the pain episode, and also tend to negate the value of the person. From specific instances, wide and condemning conclusions are drawn (e.g., "I can't peel the potatoes for supper . . . therefore I am nothing more than a worthless person"). They are unwarranted conclusions. As Flor, Behle, and Birbaumer (1993) showed, the major negative themes of the cognitions are *helplessness/hopelessness and catastrophizing*.

In addition, there is a strong tendency to *overpredict* the amount of pain that one will experience from particular activities or events (see Chapter 3).

When the pain problem persists over many months or many years, repeated negative and self-defeating thoughts and appraisals can have a pronounced effect. It is natural that such reactions will occur when pain persists long after healing. However, there are deleterious effects of letting these thought patterns continue. They tend to undermine the person's confidence and lead to increased feelings of defeat. In addition, and most important to the present session is the fact that they generate a reluctance to act or use any coping strategies that may relieve or reduce the pain problem. Needless to say, a lowering of mood and self-esteem may be aggravated by other long- or short-term problems or mishaps that occur. Again, the reactions of the family to the person's pain problem may contribute to the sufferer's growing sense of defeat.

Reducing activities and the increasing frequency of depressive or helpless thoughts may result in the sufferer withdrawing from his or her favorite leisure or pleasurable activities. This leads to a gradual erosion of all enjoyable activities, a further stimulus for increasing depression. The overprediction of pain can produce a similar retraction of activities and ensuing dysphoria.

Thus, it can be seen that in reaction to continuing pain, sufferers may become trapped into a third vicious cycle, this time between depressive mood or ruminations and pain experience. It will be remembered that in the first session the link between depression and reduced pain tolerance was described. In this session, the therapist returns to this connection in order to begin a constructive consideration of how the cycle can be interrupted.

Inappropriate Appraisals of a Pain Problem

Pain can be worsened by inappropriate appraisals of the pain problem as well as by depressive thoughts that are themselves triggered by pain episodes. Examples are useful here in order to clarify this point. Contrast the effects of two different interpretations of sharp pain in the chest, shoulder, and arm after dinner. If the sufferer interprets this pain as "I am experiencing indigestion," he or she will experience very different intensity sensations and repercussions than if he or she were to make the interpretation "I am having a heart attack." Not only are the emotional repercussions from these appraisals different, the coping strategies diverge as well (e.g., taking a cup of tea as opposed to being rushed to hospital in an ambulance).

Another example of the effect of appraisal can be illustrated by describing the effect on pain intensity of visiting a doctor. Many people have noticed that merely talking to the doctor, or even sitting in the doctor's waiting room, will lead to a reduction of the pain problem *prior* to any treatment's being suggested or undertaken. The reassurance of his or her explanations about causation and about the lack of threat may greatly reduce the level of suffering.

The therapist can bring the example closer to the chronic pain patient. Contrast the experience of a back pain patient who realizes that the pain he or she feels is due to stretching and stimulation of scar tissue with that of the patient who believes that any sharp movement will lead to a crumbling of the spine, eroding of the discs, deterioration of the back.

These examples illustrate the point that understanding pain can have a dramatic effect on its appraisal, as well as the consequent level of pain that is experienced.

The way in which a person behaves when in pain is in part a consequence of the appraisals made. The person's thoughts can amplify and enlarge the pain experience, thus inhibiting the reactions that might reduce it. When pain persists past healing, it is not a sign of injury, danger, or impending disaster. Rather, chronic pain needs to become a motivator for the use of varied strategies for the management of the aversive experience.

Thus, during this didactic period, the therapist aims to draw the attention of patients to the important role that appraisals and thoughts can play in amplifying the pain experience, reducing self-esteem, and increasing a sense of helplessness that a person may start to feel in the face of continuing pain. Such thoughts can become habitual and potent inhibitors of activities and tactics that could help otherwise reduce the severity and frequency of pain episodes. Similarly, the tendency to overpredict pain can inhibit precisely those activities that will lead to a reduction of pain.

REAPPRAISAL METHODS AND SELF-TALK (TACTIC #7)

Cognitive Methods of Modulating Pain Levels

A number of reappraisal or reinterpretation tactics can be taught to patients as methods of utilizing cognitions to limit or attenuate the pain episodes. There are large individual differences in the utility of these tactics, and patients must experiment with them to find the ones most potent for modifying their own experiences. In addition, they need to be encouraged to evolve variants of these techniques, creatively using them in a manner that best suits them.

It is important for the therapist to clarify for the patient what type of expectation he or she should have of these cognitive tactics in order to avoid disappointment and encourage frequent practice. These methods cannot be expected to prevent pain or immediately cure a continuing pain problem. They are presented to the patients as a selection of alternative tactics that may be useful in managing episodes of pain that are interfering with normal activity. Having self-monitored pain levels for some weeks, patients will know on average the intensity of the peak of pain and how long it is likely to last. They need to be encouraged to use the appraisal techniques to deal with these peak periods, in which pain may dominate their consciousness and leave them with a sense of helplessness. These techniques can be contrasted to those introduced in Session #6 which emphasized the potency of attention diversion or external focusing. In contrast, most of the techniques introduced in this session encourage the patient to experiment with reinterpretation of experience in order to minimize or trivialize it.

Their records of predicted pain, compared with the experienced pain, will illuminate their tendency to overpredict the pain, and enable them to become increasingly accurate.

Cognitive Tactics: Reappraisal of Pain

Transforming Sensation

The first technique is one of imagining the painful part of the body to be numb and anaesthetized. Various imaginative reinterpretations can be experimented with (e.g., imagining the pain area as made of rubber, or "bionic" and without sensation). Probably the most powerful use of this tactic occurs when patients develop their own personalized methods. An example of an individually derived form of this tactic is that of a patient suffering from persisting whiplash pain, who used to imagine that her shoulders and neck were made of chocolate. As she proceeded with this method she would imagine that the chocolate was becoming hot, melting, and turning smooth and liquid. As it became smooth, it flowed away from her shoulders, and she felt a reduction in pain.

Transforming Context

Another imaginative method is that of transforming the situation or context. Some people claim that they can gain relief by imagining the pain they are experiencing as appropriate for a different situation.

Such methods may be better for people with discrete bodily pains other than headaches. An example of this might be imagining that the experience being felt (e.g., in the kneecap) is a function of kneeling while scrubbing the floor or pushing a knee against a door in an attempt to open it. Thus the experience is appropriate for an imagined context in which the sensation is neither serious nor dangerous, and unlikely to produce progressive distress. For former athletes, these images can be particularly useful. They may imagine that what they are feeling is muscular strain while running, hurdling, climbing mountains, hiking, and so forth. They imagine themselves experiencing sensations that they are quite willing to withstand because of the satisfaction of the activity and the goal of success.

Denial and Redefinition

Some patients find great relief from the method of denial. In this case, they are saying to themselves that they are *not* in pain and may redescribe the experience in terms of, for example, stretching of the scar tissue, pulling of muscles, tightening of the jaw, pulsing of the arteries, and so on. There are large individual differences in the value of this technique.

Limiting the Scope of Pain

A technique that often proves of great use to patients is the idea of *limiting the pain*. They are taught to define the area in which they are feeling pain, its depth, and its spread. After enduring a chronic problem for many years, sufferers tend to enlarge its scope and feel that they are hurting all over. Carefully limiting its scope is often a useful tactic and while doing so, patients are defining the areas of their bodies that are entirely free of pain.

Relocation of Pain

This tactic, known as "relocating," asks the sufferer to try to shift his or her pain to a new location in the body (e.g., the opposite side of the body). It can be used in combination with limiting the scope of pain or on its own. This intriguing tactic has yet to be fully explored by those working in pain management. To try to move a pain from its current site appears to take great concentration. More often than not, the actual movement proves impossible. However, the concentration and attention that is necessary to try to move it can lead to a diminution of the pain. Occasionally, a patient will report success in shifting its locus, or even removing it.

Relocating Thoughts

With this tactic the sufferer shifts his or her thinking to a nonpain site. It is often a useful attention focus task for people who are reporting long periods of extreme pain and difficulty in managing the fatigue that sets in. They are asked to relocate their thinking—to concentrate their attention on an area of the body in which they feel no pain and try to center their attention on that point. Ask them to choose a site that is entirely pain-free and to fix their attention on that area. They are asked to try to "think" from that spot.

Having described these techniques to the group, induce relaxation, in a short induction method (Appendix X), and demonstrate to the patients how they may use these techniques. Go through the techniques one by one, giving patients an opportunity to experiment with the technique while remaining relaxed. The induction of relaxation acts to quieten the system and make it easier for patients to concentrate on the task being given to them. Having gone through each technique in turn, arouse the group and discuss with them the utility of these methods. Emphasize the individual differences in reaction as a further motivation for their experimentation with cognitive methods during the next week.

Problem Solving

The expectation of patients with respect to situation and effectiveness of tactics can influence their motivation to work on these techniques. Emphasis should be placed on the fact that patients can use these techniques to get periodic relief and reductions in the levels of pain they are experiencing. They are not designed to be miracle cures or long-term solutions. They are one type of tactic that a person may use to get him- or herself through peak discomfort periods, to speed the reduction of pain intensity, and to achieve a lower "trough." More broadly, they contribute to the improved cognition that they can influence their pain, that they are not entirely helpless.

Reference to the self-monitoring done by patients in the first five weeks is useful. They are now well aware that their "peaks" are relatively short in duration and that certain techniques can be useful in the rising period of pain to prevent it from reaching intolerable levels.

Many patients forget techniques explained to them during the sessions, and a written description of these cognitive techniques will prove useful. The therapist may wish to introduce a rating form, which patients can use during the week to evaluate the usefulness of these techniques at different levels of pain.

Self-Talk and the Management of Depression

Negative, exaggerated self-talk in the face of pain is such a common reaction to continuing pain problems, that it is important to offer advice to patients on how to deal with both this and the ensuing depression. The first step toward this was taken by patients in their monitoring in the previous week. This monitoring clarified the kinds of reactions they have to intense pain episodes. Patients may wish to undertake this for a further week. Try to identify the thoughts running through their minds that are closely related to pain or triggered by pain episodes. Encourage them to clarify the extent to which they tend to overreact, indulge in catastrophic projections, or formulate negative and bleak overgeneralized conclusions about themselves and their actions. In addition, encourage them to clarify the extent to which these thoughts lead to constructive pain management strategies or to inactivity and further ruminations. They may wish to star the monitored thoughts that were self-defeating and depressive.

Once they have clarified their habitual or frequent reactions in this way, it is important to encourage them to start to short-circuit or disrupt these depressed reactions in order to restore more effective ways in which they can deal with the pain episodes. At first, replacing the negative thoughts with accurate coping statements will feel clumsy to them. But as they repeatedly undertake this replacement, they will notice a shift toward much more useful thoughts that prompt coping tactics. For example, when a pain episode begins to increase, a person may find that his or her first thought is always "I can't do . . . ", or "now I won't be able to do . . . " or, even more negative "I can't do . . . so now I won't be able to do anything else." These statements express the sense of hopelessness and impotence that the person feels in the face of increasing pain. However, it can be replaced by perfectly accurate coping statements, such as "I can control my tension by relaxing my muscles and breathing evenly and steadily"; "I can manage this pain episode by focusing my attention away from it"; "I can attend to whatever I wish"; "I can continue even if I do it in a gradual and paced manner"; "I am going to focus on what I can do and ignore those things that I find difficult at the moment."

The self-talk or self-statements have a number of characteristics in common. They are all positive, factual, and realistic, and finally lead to actions likely to reduce anxiety and catastrophizing. In addition, they break through the vicious cycle that had been operating to magnify the pain experience and extend the pain problem. Needless to say, it is inadequate for the patient merely to learn the shift in self-statements. They need to follow through by undertaking the prescribed action. The self-statement "I can't" leads only to despair and withdrawal or inactivity. The new replacements are positive and also entail a prescription for action. Thus pain becomes a challenge to be dealt with, rather than a problem that the person is failing to manage. Each episode of pain can become a signal to use pain control tactics, rather than a measure of personal defeat.

Take the opportunity to remind patients of the number of different tactics that are now available for their use. The growing sense of power to battle pain and the reduction in helplessness will begin to become evident to them. It may be worth summarizing the various tactics that have been introduced to remind them of what they can use at these times.

Although the self-talk tactics are introduced to manage the reactions to pain episodes, they will be immediately recognizable to cognitive-behavior therapists who have experience in dealing with depressed patients. The replacement statements are more rational and can override the distorted judgments so often found with mood disturbances. Such cognitive techniques have been found useful in helping in the management of depressive problems.

The gradual increase in exercise and activity that has been encouraged throughout the program will, in addition, help with mood difficulties in people for whom the therapist is aware of a larger depression component. In addition, it is wise to encourage them to perform an increasing number of positive activities between sessions. Reference to their goal sheets with respect to leisure and social activities may be helpful at this stage. Patients should be asked to increase the rewarding activities they undertake each day, beginning with three to four per day and increasing them over the final few weeks of treatment. The pleasurable events need not be costly, time consuming, or complex, and should be ones that can be easily undertaken in their everyday lives (e.g., eating a favorite fruit, listening to a favorite piece of music, phoning a friend).

Problem Solving

It is important not to include in group treatment people whose depression is severe. Although their problems may be modifiable using cognitive-behavioral techniques, they will need considerable individual attention and careful monitoring, which is impossible in a group setting. They have, therefore, been excluded from this type of program (see Chapter 3 regarding exclusionary criteria). Members of the group will have levels of depression that can be adequately modified by the type of cognitive-behavioral advice offered in this chapter. The major aim of this session (Session #7) is to acquaint the patients with the link between mild or moderate depression and chronic pain so that they recognize such dysphoria as an understandable and natural consequence of their persisting pain. In addition, they are given strong motivation, and skills, to begin to resolve the vicious cycle that can develop between dysphoria and pain.

HOMEWORK ASSIGNMENTS

New Strategy Practice

This week, patients are asked to decrease their negative self-talk by replacing it, wherever possible, with a positive coping statement that they then act on. The importance of catching these negative thoughts as they occur needs to be emphasized. Patients are encouraged to use self-talk whenever they need it to reappraise and eliminate catastrophic interpretations of their pain.

They are also asked to increase pleasurable activities. For those struggling with depression, specific tasks may be needed. Encourage them to nominate one or two new activities that they will undertake during the coming week. These should be carefully defined, and group discussion is often useful in defining the assignment.

The potency of reappraisal techniques for reducing pain needs to be evaluated by each member of the group. Encourage them to start using these techniques when pain levels are relatively low. Request patients to report, at the next session, the utility of each of these techniques for their particular pain problems.

Continuing Assignments

Drugs are now being reduced to 35% levels, while exercise quotas move up. Further assertion assignments may be given to those who are strengthening their abilities to speak more directly about their needs.

Preparation Assignments

Ask members of the group to monitor the number and type of activities or situations that they find themselves avoiding during the next week. The goal is to clarify the extent to which their avoidance is due to their current levels of pain as opposed to their anticipation of the potency of certain stimuli to provoke pain; that is, the degree of accuracy of their predictions of pain. Patients who have a tendency to become overcommitted to activity and to push themselves excessively might be requested to monitor the number of activities they undertake per day rather than the number of activities they avoid. The next session will concentrate on patterns of activity and the issue of activity pacing, and this homework task forms an excellent preliminary exercise prior to undertaking this topic.

SUGGESTED READINGS

Romano, J. M., & Turner, J. A. (1985). Chronic pain and depression: Does the evidence support a relationship? *Psychological Bulletin, 97,* 18–34.

Sternbach, R. A. (1974). *Pain patients: Traits and treatment.* New York: Academic Press.

Turk, D. C., Meichenbaum, D., & Genest, M. (1983). *Pain and behavioral medicine: A cognitive behavioral perspective.* New York: Guilford Publications.

CHAPTER **14**

The Role of Activity Pacing
(Session #8)

REVIEW OF PREVIOUS ASSIGNMENTS

Following up the homework assignments from the previous session, the therapist should inquire about the difficulty or ease with which patients had been able to reduce their negative cognitions about pain and replace them with positive cognitions. If some patients have been monitoring for a further week (in order to clarify their habitual patterns), they will now be ready to begin to counteract them. Inquiries should also be made about the increase in pleasurable activities (especially in patients with a depression component to their problem).

Avoidance Patterns

For this session, the group had been asked to monitor the extent to which they avoid various activities because of pain or the belief that activity may provoke more pain (overprediction of pain). In some patients, the avoidance patterns are so well established that their lives have been drastically modified. In such cases, the avoidance may not be evident to them (e.g., people who have been out of work for years, women who now have home help, patients with facial pain who never eat crunchy foods). In addition, there is a group of patients who have a tendency to become overactive, only avoiding when the pain is totally incapacitating. These individual differences among patients in the ways they respond to pain will become evident if different members of the group are encouraged to summarize their weeks' monitoring of activity patterns.

THE ROLE OF ACTIVITY PACING AND BEHAVIORAL AVOIDANCE

Behavioral Reactions to Continuing Pain

When pain problems have persisted for months, or even years, gradual changes occur in the activity patterns of the sufferers as well as in their expectations about what they can achieve. Certain activities become associated in their minds with pain. Gradually they develop the expectations that certain types of work or activity will inevitably lead to further suffering. In the early days of a pain problem, this may well be accurate. Certain types of movement (e.g., lifting or running) and certain types of activities (e.g., concentration or social interaction) may have led to increases in pain. However, as the pain problem persists, the linkage between activities and pain increments becomes looser. However, the belief that such activities will definitely exacerbate the pain problem remains strong. There is a strong tendency to overpredict pain. When this occurs, at least two types of reactions become evident.

1. On the one hand, patients may tend to *reduce* their involvement in physical or other activities as much as possible. This occurs in order to restrict the current level of pain and to prevent it escalating as predicted. This policy can be characterized as a "wait until" policy and is probably the most common [see Figure 14.1(i)]. It is, in fact, a policy that is recommended by numbers of physicians during the early period of healing (first 72 hours) of an acute injury. Unfortunately, the patient may continue to

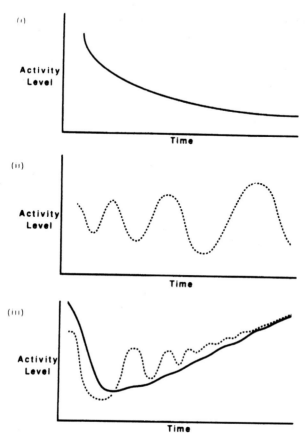

FIGURE 14.1   Activity levels.

maintain the policy even when all the healing has been completed. In addition to the deterioration in fitness and the weakening of the body that results, the frustration and depression of being cut off from normal rewards and satisfaction is considerable, setting up the vicious cycle that was discussed in the previous session.

2. An alternative reaction by some patients is to undertake even more activity despite their pain [see Figure 14.1(ii)]. These patients begin by becoming more active than they were before the injury, involving themselves in an excessive number of activities that are halted only by such severe episodes that they are no

longer able to function. They overreact. There is an intensification of activities in an unrelenting manner and a determination not to be beaten. This can lead to longer and longer periods of incapacity between activities (e.g., Arntz & Peters, 1995).

Although these two types of reactions appear to be very different, they are likely to be overlapping and may prove to be related. Patients may start off, after a short period of waiting for healing, to experiment with a return to work or activity, which may be in excess of what would be appropriate immediately posthealing. The frenetic, continuous activity is only broken up by episodes of extreme pain and collapse. As this pattern continues, the periods of collapse become longer, and finally the person is defeated and adopts an inactive style. An example of this was seen in a back pain patient who had reduced his activities to lying on the floor during the day and being fed liquid food by his wife. He had come to believe that *any* movement would exacerbate the pain he experienced!

The overactive and avoidant reactions to continuing pain are probably determined by such factors as the tendency to overpredict the pain, the personalities of the patients, their learning as children, their construal of pain, and the amounts of encouragement and reward for inactivity their families or friends give them. Patients listening to these two common reactions to pain may be able to recognize either or both tendencies in themselves. Very often, headache patients are more aware of a tendency to frenetic overinvolvement, periods broken only by severe migraines. Occasionally, chronic pain patients will report having begun with a policy of periodic overactivity that gradually changed toward the first reaction pattern (of waiting until pain recedes before undertaking activities).

Encourage different members of the group to clarify the reactions that have predominated for them, drawing out the similarities and differences among them. Although the two reaction patterns described are in many ways opposed, they both tend to increase over time and leave the person with a sense of helplessness and defeat. The person who is waiting for pain to cease (avoidant) tends to become increasingly inactive and oversensitive to stimuli. His or her reactions to stress (noise, being with other people, being under any kind of pressure) intensify, probably because these stimuli are now infrequently encountered, and are reacted to as novel stimuli. Needless to say, the person becomes unfit and is more likely to feel the effects of any type of activity. A belief is fostered, though seldom tested, that any activity will produce more pain—that is, over-prediction. Unfortunately, these people cut themselves off from diverting activities and from any chance to use attentional focusing techniques. They are often bored, intellectually unstimulated, and socially isolated. Many of their former pleasures, which they had gained through their own activities and involvements, are lost. The most likely response in such a situation is a sense of defeat, helplessness, and depression.

The results of the second type of reaction (overactivity or confrontation) overlap with the above. They tend to underpredict their pain, at first, and undertake excessive activities. This can be followed by the thought that a cessation of these activities will lead to a rebound of pain. There is little pacing of activities, little rest, and seldom any periods of relaxation. Often the endpoint of this cycle is pain that is more intense on waking and may even wake the person during the night. During the day, they keep going by excessive or even frenzied activity. As periods of relaxation are invariably associated with pain and discomfort, they are avoided. Magnified to this extent, situations that would not normally produce a great deal of reaction become stressful. These people may react to them in ways that increase their levels of arousal and make them more prone to pain episodes. Although not cut off from activities and social situations (in the way in which the first reactors were), they often suffer from periods of failure, frustration, and depression when their overcommitment is broken by periods of severe pain that halt their activities. It can be seen that, in this respect, the sense of inadequacy and frustration is similar in the two groups, although it is probably more persistent and self-defeating in the first group, who have curtailed their activity level.

Reestablishing Normal Levels of Activity

Having described these two patterns to the patients, it is important to point out that with a continuation of these patterns [see Figure 14.1(i) and (ii)] neither group will return to their prepain activity levels. However, it is possible to break through these behavioral patterns and begin to reestablish more normal levels of activity. The aim during treatment is gradually to ease each group back toward a level that approximates their prepain levels [see Figure 14.1(iii)]. For the avoidant group, this is a question of gradually undertaking more activity, repeatedly disproving that involvement and participation produce a worsening of their problems. This is facilitated by systematically recording predicted and reported pain levels. Similarly, those who have been overactive, followed by periods of underactivity, are encouraged to gradually reduce the intensity of both these reactions, bringing themselves slowly to a more reasonable, attainable level of activity. In both types, the method by which more normal activity levels are established is termed "pacing." Although this notion is introduced for the first time in this eighth session, it has been undertaken throughout the treatment program and is epitomized by the graded exercise program. Each patient's success in achieving exercise goals, or in reducing drug level, is a testament to the fact that the *gradual* approach can lead him or her further than continuing a habitual pattern that had developed.

ACTIVITY PACING (TACTIC #9)

The positive tactic of pacing activities is less discrete than the tactics introduced earlier. However, it is an extremely important one for chronic pain patients to grasp. The aim of this tactic is to encourage patients to normalize their activity levels by a procedure called "pacing."

Encourage each patient to evaluate his or her own response tendency. Has the tendency been to withdraw and wait for recovery *before* continuing plans, or has it rather been a mixture of defiance and overwork followed by collapse? Encourage patients to itemize the types of activities that they tend to avoid and those they undertake in excess. When the "avoid until" pattern dominates, patients need to be encouraged to persist with their goals *despite the pain*, using self-management strategies. Often it is easier to move toward the goal in a graded and modified form. Now possessing a number of different pain management skills, patients find this becomes feasible, and formerly unattainable goals gradually become achievable. Remind the group that new activities need to be performed in a graded and slow manner, building up the person's tolerance steadily rather than demanding prompt perfection. When the desire to avoid or withdraw occurs, the person is urged to continue despite the pain, using as many tactics as necessary.

If, in self-monitoring, patients find that they have undertaken an excessive number of activities despite the pain, "pacing" takes a different form. Rather than introducing new activities, they are working toward limiting their involvements. They can allow themselves contrasting activities to break the persistent, concentrated work (e.g., relaxation breaks, time off from activity at regular intervals, increasing physical movement and activity between tasks). Caution these patients against reacting to an improvement in their pain problems as a signal to rush back into even more intense overcommitment. Improvements in their problems can be taken as indicating that the revised approach is more sensible. The aim is to increase the amount of time that they can spend peacefully on pleasurable activities not associated with pain episodes.

When self-monitoring reveals both the "avoid until," as well as "confront despite" tendency, the pacing problem is more intriguing and challenging. It is necessary to equalize the two reactions by pacing and reducing pressure when the overactive tendency emerges, but discouraging avoidance and withdrawal when the "wait until" tendency starts to dominate. The aim is to find a level of intensity and involvement in living that does not exacerbate the pain problem but allows patients to obtain the social stimulation and involvement in life that makes it gratifying. It will take time and practice to establish the appropriate level of activity.

Problem Solving

The major problem the therapist has in this session is in drawing patients with different habitual patterns toward pain into a discussion that focuses their attention on the commonality, yet acknowledges important differences. Headache patients form a particular subgroup in this respect, and a special appendix is available with a discussion of how to integrate their needs in the discussion of activity pacing (Appendix VII).

CUE-CONTROLLED RELAXATION (TACTIC #10)

Cue-controlled relaxation is an important technique for people trying to break these habitual responses to pain. It provides them with a quickly induced, potent method of reducing pain and discomfort. It often allows them to continue an activity despite pain or to calm themselves quickly and reduce their overcommitment to a more manageable and satisfactory level. This tactic entails the induction of relaxation over a 4- to 6-minute period, using a method of induction that is an abbreviated form of the longer method taught to them in Session #2. After eight sessions of training, most patients are capable of inducing relaxation quickly, especially when they have mastered the diaphragmatic breathing. Demonstrating this technique to them during the practical section of this session makes them aware of how potent their relaxation techniques have now become. Two short induction procedures can be found in Appendix X. They teach a method of relaxing the muscles, without a tensing preliminary, on the diaphragmatic out breath, combined with self-talk.

The word *relax* or the invocation of a relaxing image can become the *cue* for a relaxation response. When relaxation induction becomes short (i.e., three to four minutes), the method can be incorporated into their daily lives. It will help eliminate the anticipatory avoidance that is often well established in chronic pain patients. Cue-controlled relaxation can also be used as a way of pacing those who have become overactive.

Induce cue-controlled relaxation two or three times for patients during this session, demonstrating that this can be done in standing or sitting positions.

Problem Solving

It is useful to encourage patients to generate their own cue which they can use when inducing relaxation. Words, thoughts, or images may be particularly powerful for patients, and they will need to experiment to find the appropriate trigger. Once identified, their continual use of this trigger when relaxing (and when breathing out) will make the trigger increasingly potent as a conditioned stimulus for a full relaxation response. Many patients report that merely breathing out to start the diaphragmatic breath can become a trigger stimulus for muscular relaxation and a sense of calm. Needless to say, once this association is well established, the patients have a potent technique available to them.

HOMEWORK ASSIGNMENTS

Activity Pacing

The specific assignment generated from this session is one to encourage patients to identify their predominant behavioral reaction and to begin to pace their activities accordingly. Those unsure about their reactions may need to monitor more carefully over the next week in order to clarify the types of situations they tend to avoid or overdo. If they are clear about their tendencies, they can be encouraged to continue despite (using self-management techniques) or to begin to reduce their overcommitments.

Evaluating Strategies

As an assignment to prepare for the next, and final, session, ask patients to evaluate all the tactics that they have been taught to date and their relative potency. This can be more easily done if they are provided with an itemized list of all the techniques that have been practiced, allowing them to indicate the relative merits of each on their monitoring sheets. An example of a tactic evaluation sheet is provided in Appendix XI. Remember to clarify with patients the meaning of each of these tactics, so that they are quite clear what is meant by each one. Encourage them to utilize each of these strategies a number of times during the week, with pain at different levels of intensity, in order to establish the utility of the tactics. Emphasize the individual differences among members of the group and the importance, therefore, of their clarifying which ones will be of continuing use to them.

Continuing Assignment

Encourage the patients to see if they can reach the exercise quotas set for them at the outset. Their drug reductions will now be to approximately 15% of their original levels. Relaxation work, if it has been done consistently, will now have reached a state of expertise, with the short cue-controlled method being as useful as the longer 20-minute induction.

Encourage patients to experiment with the cue method at any time during the day when they notice a build-up of tension or need to manage pain.

Problem Solving

Some patients will become anxious about the pending withdrawal from their drugs. Although pharmacologically the liquid will be having little effect at this stage, psychological dependence may well be present. If patients become anxious about the loss of this support, it is useful to encourage them to induce cue relaxation *after* taking each spoonful of their drugs (three to four times daily) during the last week of their use. They can then continue with this short induction at the same time of day during their first week drug-free. This can act as a bridge between drug taking and no drug taking, helping them deal with the anxiety that is sometimes elevated at times when they have been accustomed to obtaining relief. Beginning the three- to-four-times daily short relaxation inductions at this stage prepares them for the changes that will take place in the week following the last session.

SUGGESTED READINGS

Arntz, A., & Peters, M. (1995). Chronic low back pain and inaccurate predictions of pain: Is being too tough a risk factor for the development and maintenance of chronic pain? *Behavior Research and Therapy, 33,* 49–53.

Latimer, P. (1982). External contingency management of chronic pain: A critical review of the evidence. *American Journal of Psychiatry, 139,* 1308–1312.

Melzack, R. (1993). Pain: Past, present and future. *Canadian Journal of Experimental Psychology, 47,* 615–629.

Moss, R. A. (1986). The role of learning history in current sick-role behavior and assertion. *Behavior Research and Therapy, 24*(6), 681–685.

Philips, H. C., & Hunter, M. (1981). Pain behavior in headache sufferers. *Behavior Analysis and Modification, 4,* 257–265.

Philips, H. C., & Jahanshahi, M. (1985). The effects of persistent pain: The chronic headache sufferer. *Pain, 2,* 163–176.

Philips, H. C., & Jahanshahi, M. (1986). The components of pain behavior report. *Behavior Research and Therapy, 24*(2), 117–125.

Rachman, S., & Arntz, A. (1991). The overprediction and underprediction of pain. *Clinical Psychology Review, 11,* 339–355.

Wall, P. W. (1979). On the relation of injury to pain. *Pain, 6,* 253–264.

CHAPTER 15

Integration of Management Techniques (Session #9)

REVIEW OF PREVIOUS ASSIGNMENTS

Goal Achievement

Referring to the goal sheets that patients completed over two months earlier the therapist can emphasize the extent to which members of the group have been able to gradually meet their exercise and drug reduction goals. Most members of the group will have reached their exercise goals at this point, and those who are very close to it can be encouraged to undertake the last few increases prior to their final reevaluation in the subsequent week. Where difficulties have arisen, either in the drug reduction or the exercise program, patients may find themselves a little further away from their goals. In this case, the therapist needs to encourage patients to continue increasing their efforts over the subsequent weeks so that they achieve the goal for their 2-month follow-up visit. Some goals may now appear unrealistic or overambitious. However, as many goals are achieved (e.g., in terms of exercise, drug reduction, etc.), it becomes a rewarding task and a useful precursor to formulating new goal sheets.

Activity Pacing

It is useful to allow time for a discussion of the extent to which members of the group were able to begin to forestall their tendencies to either avoid or overconfront. At this stage, they will probably have characterized themselves as belonging to one or another of these classes. The therapist's aim is to encourage them to take action to modify these tendencies. Difficulties often arise in making these changes in activity pacing, and a problem-solving approach by the group can be undertaken with any patients who raise specific problems. Changing well-established habits of activity takes time and patience. In addition, these adjustments often necessitate negotiations with other members of the family or work team once the person has decided upon the changes that need to be made.

Cue-Controlled Relaxation

Check to see if patients have had any difficulties in utilizing the short induced relaxation method and whether they have begun to apply it to minimize the effects of pain on their activity. This discussion may be useful for those who have not yet begun to recognize the utility of this technique. Further practise may also be necessary if there are any people who remain unclear about the application.

Comparison of Strategies

The major aim of the therapist is to emphasize the large individual differences between the utility of the different pain management strategies. This can quickly and effectively be achieved by forming a grid on a blackboard so that each patient can sequentially indicate the efficacy for him or her of each of the methods taught during treatment. In fact, the self-monitoring instruments (used for the homework assignment; see Appendix XI) can form the basis of this grid. The therapist can thus summarize for each person his or her most useful strategies and then move on to summarize for the group the preferred methods. This approach will draw attention to the individual differences between members of the group and the variety of techniques that are now available for their use.

THE RELATIVE POTENCY OF TACTICS: A REVIEW

Summarizing The Potency of Tactics

This last session is an important one. It allows the therapist to summarize the therapy sessions, drawing the eight strands together into one fabric. This can be achieved by reminding patients of the original orientation (Session #1) and the Gate Control Model. They will have identified the physical, emotional, and cognitive influences on their pain problems and the tactics that they have discovered to exploit these influences in the modulation of pain level.

For purposes of the discussion, these tactics can be divided into those useful for the prevention of chronic pain problems and those that are better designed for immediate modulation of pain level, or what can be called *episodic control*. Examples of preventive techniques are the exercise program, relaxation work, and the reduction of drugs. Episodic control techniques are external focusing, redefinition, self-talk, and so forth. Many people find that preventive strategies can also be used for specific episodic control once they are well learned (e.g., relaxation, especially in the cue-controlled form). There is some overlap between these two types of tactics, but making this distinction helps patients formulate appropriate expectations of them. For example, exercise may, in the short-term, produce some aching and soreness, but in the long-term, produces the strengthening of muscles and return of stamina, which is a valuable insurance policy against relapse. Similarly, attention focusing will only have its impact while the person is intently undertaking this cognitive strategy. Thus, its potency lies in the episodic control of pain, not in prevention.

Choice of Tactics

The individual differences are large with respect to the utility of these tactics. Extensive research needs to be undertaken in order to clarify which chronic pain patients will benefit from which tactics. At present, it is important to encourage patients to experiment for themselves in order to pick the most relevant management techniques for their particular problem. In fact, this investigatory approach to choosing individual tactics may be an important element in this treatment approach. From the beginning, the patients are made the arbitrators of the utility of varied management techniques. They are active investigators in the cognitive-behavioral approach, rather than passive recipients of instructions. It is likely that utilizing this approach engenders large changes in self-efficacy and perceived control over pain, both of which result from this treatment approach (Philips, 1987a). By identifying the tactics that are most useful, patients can then move on to concentrate on the efficacious ones, tuning or perfecting them still further so that they become effective tools in the management of their pain problem.

It will be apparent, when filling in a separate grid for each patient, that there are tactics they have not yet tried. In this case, clarify the method again to the patients, referring them to any written material provided at that session, and encourage them to check on the value of the tactic prior to making a final decision about its importance in their repertoire. When a tactic has been tried and found ineffective, patients should be encouraged to dispense with it and to focus their attention on those tactics that have demonstrated their value. People who report that daily exercise is a useful management technique and that they have achieved the goals set by themselves or the physical therapist should be encouraged to continue at this level on their own for the two months prior to follow-up. It is important that this pattern of exercise be well established so that it persists even when they are not attending regular sessions. At the two-month point, the therapist can speak to them about the feasibility of dropping back to 3 to 4 times a week rather than the 7 times a week that they will have achieved by the end of treatment. It is often the case that preventative strategies are the ones ignored once a problem becomes less intrusive. This is understandable, as the stimulus for undertaking the strategies is reduced. However, it is worth reminding patients that they have improved in part because of these preventive strategies and that maintaining them will ensure their continuing health.

Maintaining Momentum or Counteracting Setbacks

The therapist also needs to anticipate the apprehensions of patients as they come to the end of treatment. Appropriate expectations and motivations should be suggested for the next two months, in which they are expected to utilize techniques without any direct involvement with the therapist or group. It is useful to provide them with a specific time when they will be reassessed and can discuss any difficulties or successes with the therapist. A two-month period working on their own (in other words, the same amount of time that they have had in treatment) has been found a useful interval, one that provides an appropriate goal to work toward.

Integration of Management Techniques (Session #9)

With patients who are concerned about the final reduction of medication, the emphasis should be put on the lack of potency of the tiny dose they have been on during the past few weeks. There is very little difference, physiologically, between taking the drug at 15% and not taking the drug at all. In addition, the use of skills, especially anxiety management and relaxation work, at times when they would have taken the medication, can be potent. If necessary, this last stage can be divided in half, and patients can have a 7% dose in the next week and take one extra week to reduce to 0%. However, this option should not be raised for the majority of cases; it should only be used when further negotiation with the patient indicates that he or she is determined not to eliminate the drug during that last week of treatment. It is unwise to give placebo doses. Part of the drug reduction work is to deal with the dependence on the actual ingestion of tablets, or the spoonful of liquid, associated in the past with pain relief. This dependence is as important to deal with as physiological addiction. Leaving patients on placebo doses, though producing no physiological consequences, leaves a weakness in their management of pain that can lead back into the abuse of drugs. Patients who have in the past used multiple drugs to manage pain should be warned at this time not to consider using other drugs during the next two-month period, but to do without any drugs in the management of pain.

Management of Headache Without Drugs

Some patients who have come off drugs completely may be concerned about how to manage the occasional extreme episode (as with vascular headaches). They should be encouraged at this stage to use other management techniques wherever possible rather than falling back on the drug use, which has proved detrimental to the long-term management of their pain problem.

For a small subgroup who find themselves left with periodic incapacitating migraines, the feasibility of circumscribed use of drugs to deal with infrequent episodes may need to be discussed with them. Where possible, this is best left until follow-up to allow for further reduction in migraine frequency with use of their pain management techniques. If further advice is requested at that point, advise on how to use drugs to avoid development of tolerance or toxic effects. These issues should be discussed by the therapist with the patient's GP once the program finishes, so that the physician is guided on how to handle requests for medication in a manner that reinforces the work achieved during the program.

REVIEW OF MANAGEMENT TACTICS

This practical period can be used for a brief review of the eight tactics and practice of techniques that any members of the group are having problems with or have failed to try. The emphasis in this period is upon the use of these techniques for episodic management, and thus the short cue relaxation technique can be stressed (6 minutes or less, induced using breath or imagery cues).

Encourage patients to describe any idiosyncratic tactics they have developed. Some tactics may have been modified by patients, and these changes may have made them increasingly potent. Individually derived or modified tactics may be the most useful, and any examples of these evolutions will encourage patients to become flexible in their use of the management techniques taught and to continue to evolve personalized methods. An example was provided by a patient who used the following imaginative technique to great effect: He would imagine that he was building a wall of dominoes as a barrier to the experience of pain. When he felt a surge of pain, he would imagine himself erecting his dominoes to prevent the spread and experience of pain. If pain surged forward, it would push over his dominoes, and he would imagine himself lining them up again as a defense against this "enemy." He perfected this technique and reported himself able to reset his dominoes within 3 to 4 seconds of first detecting an increase in pain.

FINAL ASSIGNMENTS

Goal Sheets

Provide the patients with new goal sheets to fill in for the next two-month period and ask them to bring the completed sheets to their person posttreatment evaluation (within the next week). Remind them again about the importance of realistic, specific, and practical goals that will move them on further toward their long-term goals.

Self-Monitoring

At this time, it will be useful for patients to fill in one more self-monitored diary, for 1 week, to allow the therapist to make an assessment of the effect of the program on their current pain levels. Many will protest about the refocusing of attention on pain, having learned the lessons of Session #6! It is praiseworthy, but in this case they must be persuaded to give the therapist a chance to see how they are currently dealing with pain, prior to returning to their external focusing approach to their problem. They may find it easier to monitor at meal times (3 times a day), thinking back over each section of the day, rather than having to keep pulling out their forms on an hourly basis.

Pleasurable Activities

Finally, encourage patients to increase the activities that bring them pleasure. The habit of refraining from undertaking too many activities is well established, and now that they are relatively pain-free and more able to handle it when it occurs, they need to be reminded of the necessity to think about enlarging their scope and feeling positive about their capacity to participate in activities that previously they had ruled out.

PART III

Outcome Evaluations

Introduction

The last part of this book concentrates on the issue of evaluations. Initially, the patient and therapist will need to clarify the stage of patients' improvement as a consequence of their involvement in a cognitive-behavioral management program. Because of the type of approach used, the two months in treatment are conceived as the beginning of the changes that will increase as skills are practiced and used. Examples of the gradual nature of change with treatment and during the follow-up period are provided to illustrate this point.

In addition to the therapist and patient evaluating the changes made, it is important for the therapist to communicate these changes to the referring physician. It is, of course, the physician who will be seeing the patient on a continuing basis and whose aid needs to be recruited in reinforcing the changes made during treatment. The more understanding the referring physician has of a psychological approach to the management of chronic pain, the better able he or she will be to handle any issues that arise and refer the patient back for booster treatment should this be required. The physician will find the job considerably easier if he or she is gradually informed about the nature of the chronic pain management and its efficacy. As a consequence, a brief review of the literature to date that evaluates the effect of a cognitive-behavioral program is included.

Finally, given the relative novelty of these techniques, clinicians are wise to involve themselves in clinical research, wherever possible, in order to clarify the therapeutic processes and increase the efficacy of the methods taught. The current program has been established to provide a service to sufferers, to encourage further research and to explore the many questions that remain unanswered with respect to pain management.

CHAPTER 16

Evaluation of the Effects of Treatment

PATIENT EVALUATION

Following the completion of the 9-week program, it is of importance for each person to meet the therapist and to discuss the effects of treatment. At this time, no further modification is attempted, but the therapist is listening in order to evaluate the change that has occurred as a consequence of the patient's exposure to this cognitive-behavioral approach.

In addition to the completion of the original questionnaires and pain monitoring methods, a modified version of the behavioral assessment questionnaire is useful in surveying the size of the remaining problem (frequency, intensity, duration of the residual problem, percentage of interference of problem on different aspects of the person's life, use of medications, if any, and behavioral avoidance).

There are considerable differences in the focus of the effect of this approach. The clinician listening to the patient at the conclusion of treatment may be more influenced by changes in some variables than others (Philips, 1987a). The questionnaires allow a wider and more independent assessment, from the patient's point of view, of the size and scope of the residual problem.

Assessment also allows comparison to be made at follow-up evaluations. The therapist may be able to recognize the patients for whom further treatment may be necessary at this stage, or to advise certain patients to seek help for associated or other psychological problems that have become apparent as the pain problem is reduced (i.e., assertiveness training, attention to anxiety management, etc.).

STAGES OF IMPROVEMENT

Against a history of many years of chronic pain, a 9-week treatment program is remarkably short. Many habits of response are present that help perpetuate the patient's difficulties. Habits are not changed suddenly but require gradual replacement with more appropriate patterns of response. When this is done, it is likely that the former behavior will be extinguished. During the 9-week treatment program, a major step is taken by patients toward shifting their habitual maladaptive behavioral response to pain and substituting more adaptive ones. As patients continue to use the skills taught to them, the new behavior will be strengthened and the therapeutic effect will increase. However, the cognitive changes tend to lag behind; they can be desynchronous (Rachman, 1990).

This pattern has been detected as a response to the treatment approach. The patient's problems have been shown to be at their lowest point 1 year posttreatment, showing a steady decline at each of the posttreatment evaluation points (1 week posttreatment, 2 months, and 12 months later) (Philips, 1987a). In assessing patients posttreatment it is important to look for the onset of therapeutic shifts in assessment measures, which may increase during the posttreatment period. If *no* changes are made during treatment, it is unlikely that they will occur spontaneously during the follow-up period. However, when a shift is seen *during* treatment, it is sensible to expect that this will increase with continuing practice of self-management techniques.

Patients come to treatment with very different histories and residual difficulties. Consequently, there will be great individual differences in the number of the changes produced during the treatment period. A number of cases will illustrate the breadth of changes made by nine patients during treatment and their subsequent progress during the follow-up period. Further research is needed to examine the process by which cognitions and behavior are shifted during the nine-week treatment period. To what extent this is a gradual, incrementing process, or if it occurs in stepwise function will be of great interest. In addition, the way in which patients integrate the techniques into their lives is intriguing. During follow-ups, it has been evident that patients increasingly adopt their methods as ways of living rather than as specific tactics to use only when faced with pain. As time goes on, they may be inclined to report no further use of the tactics, but in the descriptions of their lives, it will be evident that they have absorbed many aspects of the program and use them almost as a natural pattern within their daily life (e.g., breathing away tension when aggravated, or regular exercise).

Case Number 1

Mrs. N. was a 47-year-old woman with a 10-year history of low back problems. She reported a high level of pain and discomfort in the lower back, with occasional pinching in the left side of her hip. Her pain had a strong episodic pattern, with pain rising to 3 (0-to-5 scale) at its worst, but on average, remaining at approximately 1.5. She spoke of extensive avoidance behavior, dramatically reduced activity levels, and a curtailed social life. She reported difficulties managing her personal relationships and her work as a full-time manager. She estimated her problem to be 8 on a 0-to-10 scale on which 10 represents a major, incapacitating problem.

At the completion of the treatment period, she reported herself to have no problems, but felt she had to remain vigilant about her back. There was a dramatic drop in all of the assessment measures. She estimated the interference of pain on her life as minimal and was experiencing very low levels of pain approximately three times a week (0.47 on a 0-to-5 scale). She reported much less avoidance, and considerable success in pacing activities, and was able to undertake anything she wished to do. She was using no medication and was exercising regularly for 20 minutes a day on average.

When seen at one-year follow-up, she reported no pain at all and rated her control over her pain as being complete (10 on a 10-point scale). She was using most of the tactics on a regular basis and was particularly enthusiastic about the utility of muscular relaxation, regular exercise, activity pacing, and mental distraction. She never used drugs and was walking regularly, as well as being involved in an individual exercise program two to three times a week. The patient reported being able to do "everything except the vacuuming." She described herself as no longer thinking of herself as having a pain problem; she felt that the treatment had had a lasting effect on her management of pain and needed no further advice or treatment.

Case Number 2

Mrs. F. was referred to the service because of multiple chronic pains, which were focused in the back, knees, and elbows. She reported back pain since adolescence, but at a much more severe level in the last 5 years, since helping to cut down a tree. She had seen innumerable specialists and had had many types of treatment, including two weeks of hospitalization.

Her self-monitoring showed her to be experiencing constant pain with an average of 2.6 on a 0-to-5 scale, and she was dependent on Serax® (see Chapter 10) in order to sleep. She rated herself as having little control over her pain and felt that her problem was at a level of 7 in terms of its severity (0-to-10 rating, where 10 represents a major incapacitating problem).

There appeared to be very little activity undertaken during the day, probably because of her strong belief that any activity (e.g., housework, sex, etc.) would elicit high levels of pain. Her husband undertook most of the housework, and she spent many hours of each day resting. During flare-ups, she stayed in bed, and there were times when her husband had to carry her to the washroom. She came to the initial assessment interview in running shoes and loose clothing and had great difficulty in sitting through the assessment. She had been unable to wear heeled shoes for many years.

At the completion of treatment, she reported herself to be virtually pain-free, with no interference of pain in her activities, no use of drugs to manage her pain, including a cessation of the use of Serax to sleep, and a capacity to walk for up to 4 1/2 hours without difficulties. Test results showed a large percentage of improvement on every assessment measure. She evaluated her problem as a 3 on a 0-to-10 scale and felt that her control over the pain had reached an 8 on a 0-to-10 scale, where 10 was complete control.

At 1-year follow-up, Mrs. F. arrived for the interview in high-heeled shoes and dressed in the clothes of a professional. She reported having "very little problem to speak of." She was using no pain pills other than Feldene for her rheumatism, which she had used throughout. She was exercising daily, doing 45 minutes of the stretching and strengthening exercises given to her. She rated the average level of pain as 1.5 on a 0-to-5 scale, but experienced long periods when it was 0. The patient was using almost all of the tactics taught to her, without thinking of them, as a part of her manner of living. She felt that the treatment had had a lasting effect on her ability to manage pain. Since treatment concluded, she had completed a training course in real estate work and was employed full-time. She was successfully managing the marital difficulties produced by her return to work and reported feeling closer to her husband than she had in years.

Case Number 3

Ms. D. was a 32-year-old PhD student and part-time teacher. She had a long history of severe headaches, which had begun in her childhood, when she was approximately 12 years old. On being assessed, she reported that her headaches had gradually been worsening, especially in the 3 months prior to the treatment onset, despite multiple specialist referrals and treatments. Her 2-week monitoring showed daily headaches, with an average duration of 10.7 hours and an average intensity of 2.02 on a 0-to-5 scale. She was using Fiorinal C1/2, on average 6.6 tablets per day, plus Ativan, codeine, Dramamine®, and aspirin. Her use of drugs was almost as worrying a problem to her as her incapacitating headaches, which interfered with her work and her capacity to look after her daughter. The pattern of her headaches and the associated symptomatology was suggestive of a mixed vascular migraine and tension headache problem.

Following the completion of treatment, she had improved, with a 65% reduction in her Fiorinal use, increased perceived control over her pain problem, and a reduced rating of the size of the problem (40% reduction). She reported herself to be "the best [she] has been for ages," having been almost pain-free for 2 days in the week of reassessment and then only experiencing low intensity pain on the other days of the week. She reported no need for further treatment. The patient had established a regular exercise program and was using it daily. She was using a number of strategies taught to her on a regular basis and was benefiting particularly from regular relaxation use, activity pacing, and the exercise program.

At the 2-month follow-up, the improvements were greater. She had not sought any treatment for pain in the intervening weeks and, after ridding herself of the dependence of Fiorinal C1/2 completely, was no longer using any prescribed drugs. She sporadically used aspirin and Tylenol and was exercising 40 minutes per day (brisk walking and specific exercises). The average level of pain for the 2-week period was 0.43 on a 0-to-5 scale, representing a dramatic reduction from the pain levels prior to treatment. She estimated that her control over pain had improved by 40% and that her pain problem had reduced by 50% in its size and effect on her life.

At the 6-month follow-up, when last seen, there was no depression, all the pain measures had dropped still further, and she estimated her control over her headache problem to be 70% and its impact on her life to have dropped still further. She was considered much improved and was not requesting further help with her pain problem.

Case Number 4

Mrs. J. was a 38-year-old woman with two children who had been referred by her doctor because of chronic headache problems. She had experienced migraines since the age of 13 (approximately a 25-year chronic history), with the additional development of tension headaches occurring during pregnancy. She reported a constant headache problem, with an average intensity of 2.5 on a 0-to-5 scale. For this continuous pain, she had been using Frosst 222's. Any severe headache, she felt, would lead to a classic migraine with all the usual symptoms (visual prodromata, nausea, vomiting, loss of half her visual field, noise and light sensitivity, and blurred vision). The more intense and incapacitating headaches were occurring three times a week and had led her to use and become physiologically and psychologically dependent on Fiorinal C1/2. Self-monitoring over a 2-week period prior to the onset of treatment showed her to use an average of eight Fiorinals on a bad day. She reported a strong family history of classical migraine, with her maternal grandmother, mother, and sister all being migraine sufferers.

There was some suggestion that the frequency of the migraine episodes had reduced somewhat over the years, but that the tension headaches had remained constant.

Mrs. J. made remarkable progress during the 9-week treatment program, reducing the frequency and duration of her headache problem. The continuous pattern of headaches had been broken, although daily headaches were still evident at a lower intensity level (0.3 on a 0-to-5 scale). Medication had been reduced by 55%, and her control over her problem had increased by 50% in her own estimation.

Two months following treatment, she reported herself as "feeling wonderful." She had stopped using Fiorinal C1/2 on a regular basis, and in fact reported having used only two in the two months prior to her follow-up, although she was using the occasional Frosst 222. The pattern of continuous headache had been broken and she no longer woke with headaches each day. Severe headaches had become rare. She returned to her work as a part-time stewardess.

One year after the completion of treatment, she reported that she had not seen any other professionals about her headache problem and was still using many of the tactics taught to her during her treatment program. Her headaches were still occurring daily, and she had returned to the use of Fiorinal C1/2, although at a lower level than previously (1 to 2 tablets per week maximum). She was using Frosst 222's daily, and reported headaches occurring daily, with no pain-free days in the seven days prior to this reassessment. She had developed no other problems and reported the intensity of pain to be low (1.5 on a 0-to-5 scale, on average). The patient appeared to have clarified many of the issues pertaining to her headaches and pinpointed the relationship with her husband as being a difficult one that had yet to be resolved. She was enjoying her job, her children, and her work and reported herself as being "very happy with [my] material surroundings." Although there was an indication of many of the indices of her pain problems being improved from her pretreatment levels, there was, nonetheless, evidence at 1-year follow-up of a slight loss of control. Booster sessions were suggested.

Case Number 5

Ms. W. was a 23-year-old woman with a chronic headache problem. She was severely depressed when referred and had high levels of pain of a migraine variety, localized over the right eye, particularly severe during her menstrual cycle, and associated with visual prodromata, blurred vision vomiting, and cold hands. In addition, she experienced a bilateral frontalis pain that spread from the forehead to the back of her head and down her neck. Her headache pains were constant, but markedly worse upon wakening. The tension-like headache rated an average of 6 on a 10-point scale and occurred daily, worsening through the day. The migrainous pain, when present, averaged at 6 on a 10-point scale, but was more incapacitating. Although working full-time, she reported great interference of her pain with her social life (70%), sexual activity (50%), as well as markedly reduced physical activity and concentration at work. She was severely depressed (Beck Depression Inventory = 32). Although not using prescribed drugs, she used up to twelve 222s a day, drank eight cups of coffee or tea, and was on the contraceptive pill.

As a prerequisite for inclusion in the treatment group, she was withdrawn from her oral contraceptive and was reassessed 6 months later. There was little change in any aspect of her pain problem, and in the two weeks prior to treatment, her average pain level was 3.01 on a 0-to-5 scale, with an average duration of 16.4 hours daily. She was using an average of 16 Frosst 222s, 4 Tylenols®, and 8 aspirin per day. She estimated her problem to be 8 on a 0-to-10 scale, where 10 is a major incapacitating problem, and her control to be 3 on a 0-to-10 scale, where 10 is complete control.

Following treatment, there were a number of signs of improvement. For the first time, she was enjoying many occasions of waking pain-free in the morning. She rated her average pain to be 2.5 on a 0-to-5 scale, with peaks of 4 for migraine. She was reporting 2 to 3 pain-free hours each day, and a drop in pain intensity and quality was evidenced on the McGill Pain Questionnaire, as well as a dramatic reduction in pain behavior and complaint levels, life impact. The rated control over pain had increased

40%, while the problem size had reduced 40%. She was no longer using any medication to manage pain. In addition, her depression scores had dropped to the mild level on the Beck Depression Inventory. Although still troubled with a headache problem five to six days out of seven, her migraines were occurring only once a month.

When seen one year posttreatment, she reported her perceived control to be still better, rating it 8 on a 0-to-10 scale, and rated the problem size to be 2 on a 0-to-10 scale (reduction, 60%). Her Beck Depression Inventory was normal (Beck = 8), and there were improvements on all measures assessed, particularly pain behavior, Life Impact Checklist, and the McGill Pain Questionnaire. Frequency of headache was two in every seven days, but the pain never reached a high enough level to interfere with work, concentration, or social life. At most, it appeared to reach a 2 on a 0-to-5 scale. She was exercising regularly using techniques taught to her as a part of her everyday life, and felt no need for further help.

Case Number 6

Ms. O. was a 34-year-old mother of three young children, referred by an orthopedic surgeon for evaluation of a chronic back pain problem prior to considering a second operation. Her difficulties began when she was a girl of 17, with classic migraine episodes. Her back pain problem started after the birth of her first child, 10 years prior to her coming to the clinic. She reported a marked exacerbation of her headache problem when she experienced flare-ups of her neck and back problems. Her pain problems had become worse since 1982 after her third discogram. She had consulted numerous specialists, been treated with many drugs, and became dependent upon Fiorinal C1/2 over the last 2 years. She used from 8 to 10 per day, but the average (estimated from her self-monitoring) was 6.4 tablets per day. In addition to the Fiorinal, she would go to the hospital for Demerol injections on occasion. This was not a frequent event, but nonetheless was a feature of her pain management. Her pain problem led to a dramatic withdrawal from activities, work, and home responsibility. She demanded constant attention from her husband, children, and therapist. There appeared to be long-standing social and marital problems.

Ms. O. received 12 sessions of individual pain management, after which she reported herself to be feeling completely well 75% of the time and estimated that she could now deal with the pain episodes that occurred approximately every 14 days. They were predominantly on the left side of the head, beginning at the upper neck. Her migrainous pain was as intense as previously, but less frequent and of much shorter duration. She rated her remaining problem as 4 on a 0-to-10 scale and estimated her control to have risen to 8 on a 0-to-10 scale. There were dramatic changes in her behavior, with much reduced avoidance and complaint and a complete cessation of the use of Fiorinal C1/2. Daytime resting had dropped to zero and her sleep had normalized. Her daily routine included a half hour of walking and the use of many cognitive-behavioral techniques that she had learned.

Her orthopedic surgeon, on seeing her posttreatment, reported her to still have a "degenerative C6-7 disc problem, but generally handling the offshoots very well." He wrote, "we do not know if she will always be well with respect to her neck, but certainly her response to pain will be much more satisfactory. I anticipate seeing her again in the fall and will welcome her back if she has any ongoing difficulties. She certainly seems to be a different person than when we first started out with her." Surgery, which had been pending, was canceled.

She decided to return to work on a part-time basis and, at that time, had a return of some of her pain difficulties. She was seen again during that period and proved to be very adept at using the pain management techniques. At the end of her booster sessions, she rated her control over pain as 9 on a 0-to-10 scale, achieved pain-free days, and found her migraines were associated much more clearly with menstruation. The length of difficult episodes were shortened, and apart from the menstrual migraine, her pain level was, on average, 1.5 on a 0-to-5 scale, dropping, as she used her techniques, to 0. She was not using any drugs to manage her pain, exercised daily, and had returned to full-time work.

Case Number 7

Ms. A. was referred with a 10-year history of recurrent pain focused in the upper jaw, spreading down to the chin and up to the ears and temple. She related the onset to an occasion when she bit into an apple and felt a cracking and painful sensation in her jaw on the left side. Throughout a 10-year period, the problem had a tendency to flare up every two to three weeks, but was somewhat dependent on the amount of jaw action.

She had had one long period of freedom from pain following an orthopedic surgeon's manipulation, but it had returned after a motor vehicle accident in which the left side of her face was damaged. Her present problem had occurred two years prior to the referral with the removal of a wisdom tooth. The pain became progressively worse over the two years. She was experiencing phasic and dramatic increases in pain, at which time her jaw "seemed to lock."

When assessed, she was using an average of 3.8 Robaxin® and a morphine pain cocktail. Her score was normal on the Beck Depression Inventory, and her average rated intensity of pain was 3.8 on a 0-to-5 scale. The pain was constant, and she rated her problem as 6 on a 0-to-10 scale, where 10 represents an incapacitating problem. However, she reported the problem to have a minimal impact on her life, and her levels of avoidance and complaint were low despite the high rating she had given to the size of the problem.

In addition to the jaw problem, there was some suggestion of a migraine-type headache problem, which related directly to her menstrual cycle. She was, however, not seeking help for this but was primarily interested in modifying her facial pain.

After attending an individual course of pain management, she reported that she no longer had pain in her jaw, but merely a "slight tightness on the left side." She experienced very occasional headaches, and no longer felt that her jaw was a problem; she was delighted at her success in learning how to cope with it. Self-monitoring showed no pain during the two weeks prior to the assessment, and no use of any drugs. She estimated her problem to be 0 on a 0-to-10 scale and her control to be 9 out of 10. She was eating normally and had begun to enjoy steaks and apples after a long period during which she had been unable to eat them.

At the two-month follow-up she remained pain-free and confident of her ability to manage the pain problem. All her questionnaire measures were 0. This pattern continued to the one-year follow-up, when she reported no difficulties of any sort and a control of 10/10 over her pain problem.

It is of interest to note in this case, particularly with the dramatic shift from a pain to nonpain state, that two months following the 1-year follow-up, a letter was received from this patient's oral physician, who wrote that she had reported a pain focused on dentition, as opposed to facial muscular pain or temporomandibular joint pain. A new dentist had then undertaken an extraction of her remaining upper teeth. She reported to her oral physician that her new dentures provided a great improvement in her pain problem! This would suggest that although her facial problem had been resolved, she developed a pain problem with respect to her teeth, which became the focus of her concerns and presumably led her to persuade a specialist to do further dental work. This was undertaken approximately two months after her report to our clinic that she no longer needed any help in managing her pain, and her questionnaire results showed complete control over pain. The process by which pain developed or the reasons for her failure to report it are unclear. However, it might be wise to recognize the instability of improvement in cases where there is a sudden and dramatic shift rather than a gradual improvement and development of control. In addition, this case highlights the importance of good communication links between the therapist and physicians continuing the management of the patient.

A small percentage of cases are not affected by this program. As yet, we are not able to identify these patients in advance, or explain these failures, but future research will be directed to clarifying the predictive factors. Two patients who did not improve in the program are described. The second case illustrates the importance of excluding patients who are involved in compensation cases.

Case Number 8

Ms. T. was a 48-year-old woman who was referred to the clinic for treatment of a lower back pain, which had led her to remain for long periods in bed, in response to the extreme pain in the lower back, right leg, and left leg. She had worked as a heavy machine operator until two years prior to the assessment, having stopped because of her back pain. Her pain problem had begun five years earlier. In monitoring her pain levels, it was evident that the pain was continuous, with an average intensity of 3.9 on a 0-to-5 scale. She reported attacks every two to three weeks in which the level of discomfort rose more dramatically. She had reduced all physical activity and was using an average of 1.2 Darvon and 2 diazepam daily. She evaluated her problem to be 8 on a 0-to-10 scale, where 10 is an incapacitating problem, and her control to be 5 on a 0-to-10 scale. Her depression level was moderate on the Beck Depression Inventory at the onset of treatment.

She attended all the treatment sessions, but at the end of the 9-week period there was no change in her pain problem. There was a small but insignificant change in avoidance and a larger change in her cognitive evaluation of pain, but overall, the picture had not changed significantly. Her pain remained continuous and at the same intensity level, and her use of Darvon and diazepam continued unchanged. An exercise program had never been established consistently, although at times during the nine weeks she had been able to manage walking for 15 minutes in a day.

At the two-month follow-up, the picture was much the same, with no significant changes in any of the measures taken. There was a further decline in her perceived control of her pain problem (3 on a 0-to-10 scale).

Case Number 9

Mr. C. was a 44-year-old married man referred to the clinic with an incapacitating pain problem that had led to his retirement from a job as a hotel consultant, which he had held for 20 years. He had been increasingly disabled by the pain over the two years prior to coming to the clinic. His wife worked part-time to maintain the family, and he was doing some consulting work from home.

He described his problem as constant pain in the base of the skull and in the back of his neck. He also reported pains in his legs and the right side of his body. He also suffered from daily headaches, which he felt were focused on the top of his head, and he presumed that they developed from his severe neck pain.

Mr. C.'s problems had begun three years prior to his referral when he fell from a horse onto his head and shoulders. Since that time, the pain problem had gradually worsened despite multiple and varied treatments.

At the end of the nine-week treatment program, he described himself as still having the same, if not worse, neck pain problems, with sharp pain aggravated by activity. Although attending all the sessions regularly, he made it clear that he felt most of the issues being discussed were not entirely relevant to him and that he had already achieved many of the goals the other members were working toward. He did use many of the tactics, but often tried to undermine the participation of other members of the group.

One week after the completion of his posttreatment assessment, which showed a remarkable constancy in every aspect of his pain problem, a letter was received from a group of solicitors representing Mr. C. in a personal injury lawsuit, which was to come to trial within the month. He had refrained from revealing to the therapist his involvement in the lawsuit and this fact had not been mentioned by the referring physician.

His involvement in the treatment program was, therefore, inappropriate, given the exclusionary criteria, and is an interesting testament to the importance of excluding people involved in this type of legal action.

DOCTOR/THERAPIST COMMUNICATION: PATIENT PROGRESS

If a patient returns one month or so after treatment with a resurgence of pain, a GP, however well his or her intentions, may advise bed rest and complete cessation of activity. This will undermine the progress made during treatment and the self-management approach taught.

Of particular importance for the continuing management of patients is the communication of the result of treatment to the referral source. The GP or other physician caring for the patient in the future will need to understand the type of changes that the person is trying to make and to continue to reinforce a similar approach. This is of particular importance if the patient has a setback during the post-treatment period. An uninformed physician can undermine a program if he or she is unaware of the tactics taught or of the changes that the person has already made toward returning to a normal life and leaving behind the tendency to adopt an invalid role.

The changes evident in the questionnaires are a useful means of communicating the *type* of improvement made by patients. If the therapist has been able to clarify the nature of related or unrelated psychological problems, he or she can communicate this to the referring source and make suggestions on the type of treatment that could be useful (e.g., assertion training).

DOCTOR/THERAPIST COMMUNICATION:
CHRONIC PAIN MANAGEMENT

In discussions with the referring physicians and contributing professionals (pharmacist, physical therapist), the therapist may need to serve an educative role, teaching the background to the cognitive-behavioral approach to pain management. Physicians referring regularly to the psychologist will become increasingly efficacious in their approach to pain management as they see its utility for their patients, and learn its methodology. Subsequent referrals will be of patients with more appropriate expectations and medical support.

CHAPTER 17

Concluding Notes on the Efficacy of Psychological Treatments: Research Evaluations

There is convincing evidence that psychological treatments are capable of producing significant improvements among patients with particular types of chronic pain (Flor, Fydrich, & Turk, 1992; Pearce, 1983; Tan, 1982; Turner & Chapman, 1982; Turner & Romano, 1990; Weisenberg, 1987). The most significant advances have been made in the management of chronic headache, low back pain, and the relief of postoperative pain. Useful progress has also been made in developing methods to relieve cancer pain, pelvic pain, and facial pain (Fernandez & Turk, 1989; Jensen, Turner, & Romano, 1994; Pearce, 1983; Turner & Romano, 1990).

In a meta-analytic review of 65 studies of treatment efficacy for chronic back pain, Flor, Fydrich, and Turk (1992) concluded that multidisciplinary treatments, which included psychological therapy, produced significant and enduring clinical improvements. The benefits were extensive and included reductions in pain reports and pain behavior, and improved mood and work activities. Comparable conclusions were reached by Holroyd and Penzien (1990) in their metaanalysis of headache treatment (see also Blanchard et al., 1980, 1982).

Although these analyses provide encouraging support for the use of multidisciplinary treatments for chronic pain, the quality of much of the research is wanting (e.g., poorly chosen or absent control groups), and very few of the studies enable one to isolate the particular contribution made by the psychological component of the treatment. It can be argued, however, that as virtually all modern treatment programs are integrated, multidisciplinary and multicomponent, the isolation of one or more components is often impossible and always inadvisable. The present Pain Management Program contains several interlocking components and is deliberately, necessarily, multidisciplinary. Therefore, a true evaluation of its effects can only be carried out on the full Program, with all of its parts and all of its players.

The foundation for this Pain Management Program was established over a number of years in which referrals from within and without a large general hospital were dealt with on a case by case basis. Gradually we formed a structure for the Program and a dependable collection of assessment and treatment procedures. Finally, the full Program was put to the test in a controlled evaluation of the treatment. The results were encouraging. This Program, now updated by the addition of a stronger cognitive component, was the result of clinical experiences supported by a controlled scientific evaluation.

The effects of the Program were evaluated in 1987 in the form of a control group treatment study of 40 chronic pain patients (back, head, and other pain problems). Twenty-five patients were allocated to treatment groups of 5–7 people and assessed before and after a 9-week outpatient treatment program. Follow-up evaluations were taken at eight weeks and at one year. Fifteen comparable patients (controls) accepted for treatment were placed on a waiting list; they were evaluated using similar instruments before and after their waiting period (2–6 months).

The results showed a significant clinical improvement in 83% of the treated cases and no change in the waiting list controls. The improvements appeared to be largely a function of significant reductions in pain avoidance behavior, affective reaction to pain, and depression, and a major attitude shift in respect to perceived control over pain. Changes produced by treatment endured for up to one year follow-up. In addition, important shifts in the correlations between the measures of the pain problem occurred. A growing unification of pain response occurred as the problem became more circumscribed. No differences were seen between different pain types in their response to the behavior program.

Most of the psychological methods such as the original for the present program, were spawned by behavior therapy and retain behavioral exercises and retraining as core elements in the pain management program. In keeping with the cognitive revolution in psychology, pain management programs now incorporate cognitive elements and most contemporary programs, including this Revised Program, emphasize the importance of identifying the patients' key cognitions and their role in sustaining or inhibiting the pain.

> The rationale for applying cognitive-behavioral treatment strategies to both acute and chronic pain problems is that learning new cognitive and behavioral responses to pain and stress can give the individual a sense of control over pain and decrease negative emotions, thoughts, and judgments related to the pain; this in turn, may reduce pain, suffering, and pain behavior. (Turner & Romano, 1990, p. 1711)

Cognitive-behavioral techniques, in common with all psychological pain-reducing procedures, form part of a broad, comprehensive interdisciplinary pain management program. In addition, specialized techniques, such as biofeedback, have been tried and tested with some success. In a related enterprise, significant advances have been made in developing psychological procedures that reduce the pain and distress caused by invasive and other uncomfortable medical procedures (Hathaway, 1986; Suls & Wan, 1989).

EARLY INTERVENTION

The case for early intervention is supported by the findings from a study of the evolution of chronic back pain problems. A sample of 117 patients was assessed within two weeks of the onset of acute back pain, reassessed three months later, and again after six months had elapsed from the time of onset. In this way it was possible to trace the evolution of a chronic pain problem (Philips & Grant, 1991a). A surprisingly large number of patients were still reporting significant pain at six months, thereby qualifying for a diagnosis of chronic pain (40%). In approximately 20% of all the cases, the pain reported at six months was moderate to severe intensity but only three of the total sample were still unable to work at the end of the six-month study period. Most of the changes that took place in the pain (cognitive, behavioral, and subjective) occurred within three months after onset. Thereafter the pain problem demonstrated remarkable stability. In general, the quality of the pain reported among the chronic sufferers at the 6-month point were remarkably similar to the pain qualities described at the point of onset. Contrary to expectation the psychological qualities of the pain did not undergo any significant alterations in the 6-month period.

The results of the study indicated that at least in this type of acute back pain, the crucial interval occurs between the point of onset and 3 months, during which period the greatest changes in pain take place. After the 3-month point the pain stabilized. More people were vulnerable to persisting pain than had been expected and the period of recovery was slower than anticipated. The similarity of the pain qualities at onset and at 6 months show that this type of chronic pain is best thought of as a persistence of the original acute pain experience, rather than a new or transformed pain. The period of greatest malleability is 0 to 3 months, and it is probable therefore, that psychological and other therapeutic interventions are likely to have their greatest impact within 3 months of the onset of the problem. Early intervention is recommended.

The patients who continued to report pain at the 3-month assessment period were significantly different (at the acute stage) from those patients who had largely recovered within 3 months of onset. The patients with persisting pain reported greater levels of pain at the acute stage, significantly more negative cognitions about the pain, higher anxiety, and greater disruption of their life as a result of the pain. The best predictions of chronic status were made on the basis of the patient's condition at 3 months, when 80% were correctly classified. The predictions of an absence of chronic pain were more accurate than the predictions for continuing pain; that is, patients who no longer had significant pain three months after the onset of the acute pain were extremely unlikely to report pain at the six-month reassessment point (Philips & Grant, 1991a). A single session of psychological counseling appeared to increase behavioral exercises; 63% of the patients who received the counseling were carrying out graded exercises at the 6-month point versus only 20% among the patients who were not given counseling.

Similar results were reported by Linton, Hellsing, and Andersson (1993) who studied the fate of 198 patients seeking help for acute back or neck pain. Those patients who were given early active treatment, as opposed to the usual form of treatment in which a delay of up to 10 days is common, did significantly better over the long run than did the patients who waited. "The risk of developing chronic (greater than 200 sick days) pain was eight times lower for the early activation group. This investigation shows the relatively simple changes in treatment result in reduced sickness absenteeism for first-time sufferers only. Consequently the content and timing of treatment for pain appear to be crucial. Properly administered intervention may therefore decrease sick leave and prevent chronic problems" (p. 353). The general case for taking preventive actions is set out by Linton (1985).

TRENDS

All of these developments have served to increase the optimism and enthusiasm of therapists attempting to help patients deal with their pain problems, and thousands of patients have benefited from the use of these techniques (e.g., the Flor, Fydrich, & Turk [1992] metaanalysis alone encompassed 3,089 patients with chronic back pain). The extremely welcome advances should not obscure the fact that we still lack definitive evidence to support the rationale on which these techniques are based, and that in numerous controlled trials the specific psychological techniques have been found to be as effective, but no more effective, than general, nonspecific procedures such as relaxation training. For example, in their extensive review Blanchard and Ahles (1990) found few convincing examples of trials in which biofeedback procedures were clearly superior to credible relaxation training procedures. There are, of course, powerful and pervasive nonspecific therapeutic influences in all forms of psychological therapy (Rachman & Wilson, 1980), and pain-reduction procedures are no exception. Indeed, many of these nonspecific influences can usefully be construed as evidence of cognitive influences in the experience of pain, and recruited to provide theoretical support for the introduction of cognitive elements into previously behavioral approaches to pain management. The rationale set out by Holzman and Turk (1986), with its emphasis on introducing optimism, active patient participation, promoting self-efficacy, and self-attribution of change, can easily be turned to accommodate many of the nonspecific factors that are known to contribute to therapeutic improvement.

As mentioned earlier, the evaluation of psychological techniques is complicated by the fact that they almost invariably comprise part of an integrated, multidisciplinary pain management program, and hence it is difficult to extract and evaluate the *specific* contribution made by the psychological component. Another impediment to clean, precise evaluation arises from the fact that the psychological program leans heavily on the patient's cooperation in carrying out the homework exercises, and there is no easy and reliable way to assess the extent to which patients adhere to the exercises. The assessment of the effects of the cognitive components of the treatment present additional problems, such as the timing of the cognitive changes, and their causal connection to the reductions in pain (Rachman, 1993).

It is not uncommon for therapeutic procedures to advance ahead of theoretical understanding, and given empirical support, there is every reason to use these techniques. However, enthusiasm and application should be tempered by a recognition that the theoretical justification for particular psychological techniques is lacking and therefore a source of intellectual uneasiness. There remains an urgent need to develop a broad psychological rationale for treatment and to integrate within the framework provided by the gate control model.

SUGGESTED READINGS

Anderson, T. P., Cole, G. M., Gorlickson, G., Hudgens, A., & Roberts, A. H. (1977). Behavioral modification of chronic pain: A treatment program by a multi-disciplinary team. *Clinical Orthopaedics Related Research, 129,* 96–100.

Aronoff, G. M., Evans, W. O., & Enders, P. L. (1983). A review of follow-up studies of multi-disciplinary pain units. *Pain, 16,* 1–11.

Blanchard, E. W., & Andrasik, F. (1982). Psychological assessment and treatment of headache: Recent developments and emerging issues. *Journal of Consulting and Clinical Psychology, 60,* 6859–6879.

Blanchard, E. W., Andrasik, S., Ahles, T. A., Teders, S. J., & O'Keefe, D. M. (1980). Migraine and tension headache: A meta-analytic review. *Behavior Therapy, 11,* 613–631.

Chapman, S. L., Brennan, S. F., & Bradford, I. A. (1981). Treatment outcome in chronic pain rehabilitation programs. *Pain, 11,* 255–268.

Dolce, J. J., & Crocker, M. F. (1986). Exercise quotas, anticipatory concern, and self-efficacy expectancies in chronic pain: A preliminary report. *Pain, 24*(3), 355–365.

Gottlieb, H., Streit, L. C., Koller, R., Maderasky, Z., Hockersmith, V., Kellman, M., & Wagner, J. (1977). Comprehensive rehabilitation of patients having chronic low back pain. *Archives of Physical Medicine Rehabilitation, 58,* 101–108.

Guck, T. P., Skultety, F. M., Meilman, P. W., & Dowed, E. T. (1985). Multidisciplinary pain center follow-up study: Evaluation with a no-treatment control group. *Pain, 21*(3), 295–307.

Hawton, K., Salkovskis, P., Kirk, J., & Clark, D. (Eds). (1989). *Cognitive behavior therapy for psychiatric problems.* Oxford: Oxford University Press.

Holroyd, K. A., & Penzien, D. B. (1990). Pharmacological versus non-pharmacological prophylaxis of recurrent migraine headache: A meta-analytic review of clinical trials. *Pain, 42,* 1–13.

Jensen, M. P., Turner, J. A., & Romano, J. M. (1994). Correlates of improvement in multi-disciplinary treatment of chronic pain. *Journal of Consulting and Clinical Psychology, 62,* 172–179.

Melzack, R. (1983). *Pain measurement and assessment.* New York: Raven Press.

Melzack, R., & Wall, P. (1988). *The challenge of pain.* Harmondsworth, Middlesex, England: Penguin Books.

Newman, R. I., Seres, J. L., & Yossep, L. P. (1983). Multi-disciplinary treatment of chronic pain: Long-term follow-up of low back pain patients. *Pain, 4,* 283–292.

Pearce, S. (1983). A review of cognitive/behavioral methods for the treatment of chronic pain. *Journal of Psychosomatic Research, 27*(5), 431–440.

Philips, H. C. (1987a). The effects of behavioral treatment on chronic pain. *Behavior Research and Therapy, 25,* 365–378.

Philips, H. C. (1987c). Avoidance behavior and its role in sustaining chronic pain. *Behavior Research and Therapy, 25,* 273–280.

Philips, H. C. (1988). Changing chronic pain experience. *Pain, 32,* 165–172.

Roberts, A. H., & Reinhardt, L. (1980). The behavioral management of chronic pain: Long-term follow-up with comparison groups. *Pain, 8,* 151–162.

Saunders, S. H. (1983). Component analysis of behavioral treatment program for chronic low back pain. *Behavior Therapy, 14,* 697–705.

Seres, J. L., Paynter, J. R., & Newman, R. I. (1981). Multi-disciplinary treatment of chronic pain at the Northwest Pain Centre. I. L. Lornez & K. Ng (Eds.), *New approach to chronic pain: A review of multi-disciplinary pain clinics and pain centres* (NIDA Research Monograph No. 36). Washington, DC: U.S. Government Printing Office.

Stenn, P. G., Mothersill, K. J., & Brooke, R. I. (1979). Biofeedback and cognitive behavioral approach to the treatment of myofacial pain dysfunction syndrome. *Behavior Therapy, 10,* 29–36.

Swanson, D. M., Maruta, D., & Swenson, W. M. (1979). Results of behavior modification in the treatment of chronic pain. *Psychosomatic Medicine, 41,* 55–61.

Turk, D. C., & Rudy, T. E. (1987). Towards a comprehensive assessment of chronic pain patients: A multiaxial approach. *Behavior Research and Therapy, 25,* 237–249.

Turner, J. A., & Chapman, C. R. (1982). Psychological interventions for chronic pain: A critical review, 1 and 2. *Pain, 12,* 1–46.

APPENDIX I

Description of Medication-Reduction Regime

This is an example of the type of material that can be sent to referring physicians to explain a medication-reduction program. It can be personalized and adjusted to meet the needs of a particular chronic pain clinic or psychology department.

The majority of patients with chronic pain problems are on some form of narcotic/barbiturate analgesic preparation. It is essential that patients' medication be reduced gradually and under close supervision. In order for a gradual reduction to take place, it is desirable to change to a liquid equivalent of their current analgesic medication as a first step. Some of the combination analgesic products (e.g., Fiorinal C1/2) are unsuitable for compounding in liquid form, and barbiturates or narcotics may be substituted. Equi-analgesic doses are determined and dispensed.

In addition to changing to equivalent liquid medication, the average daily consumption of analgesic is determined and given on a regular rather than on an "as needed" basis. The time-linked medication regimen (as opposed to pain-linked) is a useful second step in treatment. As the patient progresses with treatment, reductions in medication dosage will occur. The average reduction is approximately 10% to 20% per week and is determined by the progress the patient is making in the self-management of pain and his or her personal desire to reduce the medication. If the patient has difficulty at any point, the rate of reduction is slowed down. A standard reduction program that most patients are able to follow is described later. In all reductions, the volume of liquid medication remains constant while the active analgesic content is gradually reduced. Patients are requested to discontinue all other analgesic medication and to obtain their prescriptions only from the pharmacist. Your support on this issue will be much appreciated. It has been found much easier to control some of the complications of dealing with highly dependent chronic pain patients if a single pharmacy deals with all drugs; thus the general practitioner is, during the period of the pain management program, freed from his or her responsibilities for managing the medications. This is left to the physician consultant and the pharmacist, and is undertaken at the speed felt appropriate by the patient and the therapist.

To facilitate the gradual reduction of analgesic medication, the following method has been developed: After the patient has been found suitable for treatment and written consent for treatment has been received, the pharmacist will obtain a medication history from the patient. During this interview, the patient's current drug regimen will be delineated. The patient will be requested to chart all doses of analgesics consumed over a 2-week period. The patient will also be told about the need to change to a liquid equivalent medication, and any concerns will be discussed at this time (e.g., intolerance to alcohol precludes the use of elixirs, etc.). The therapist will discuss with you and the physician consultant any recommendations for equivalent liquid medication.

When treatment begins, the patient will begin taking the liquid medication on a regular basis at the dosage level of his or her most recent analgesic regimen. Following this initial stabilization period, gradual reductions in the medication will occur weekly. The standard reduction regimen used in the program is outlined below:

Week	% of Original Dose
1–2	100
3	90
4	75
5	55
6	35
7	15
8	0

APPENDIX II

Specific Flexion Exercises

The following list of general exercises may be a useful resource for psychologists who do not have physical therapy support for the establishment of an person exercise program for particular patients. The selection of the exercises for a person can be guided by the locus of their pain problem and the muscle weaknesses that they have. Head pain sufferers can be aided by encouraging them to undertake some of the exercises grouped in Sections 1 (a through c) and 5. Always remember to encourage patients to start at a very low level and to gradually increase up to approximately 10 repetitions per day. Those exercises of flexion marked with an asterisk (*) are particularly useful for mid- and low-back problems.

1. Lying on the floor, knees bent, one very thin pillow under head and neck:
   (a) Roll head gently side to side.
   (b) Tuck chin in, press back of head onto pillow gently.
   (c) Shrug shoulders up to ears.
   (d) Clasp hands, bend elbows, stretch hands up to ceiling.
   (e) Clasp hands, bend elbows, stretch arms above head.
   (f) Bend arms, punch alternate arms above head.

(g) Shrug shoulders and tighten facial muscles as you breath in deeply. Relax as you breathe out.

(h) Tighten stomach muscles, press small of back onto floor (pelvic tilt).

(i) With pelvis tilted, pull one thigh to your chest then straighten leg in the air.

(j) With pelvis tilted, straighten one leg, pull other toward your chest.

(k) With pelvis tilted, lift head and shoulders to look at knees.

(l) With pelvis tilted, sit half way up to touch knees with hands.

(m) Sit up any way you can, then lie down slowly (no arms).

(n) Sit-ups.

(o) Lift backside in the air.

2. Sit up, legs out in front of you slightly bent:

(a) Sit up straight, tuck fists into armpits, bend side to side.

(b) Stretch hands to reach feet.

(c) Bend one knee, lean over straight.

3. Lying on your side, lower leg bent:

(a) Clasp ankle of upper leg, pull it behind you.

4. Lying on your stomach (pillow under stomach):

(a) Bend alternate knees.

(b) Lift head and shoulders off bed.

(c) Lift alternate legs.

5. Sitting upright: (particularly useful for upper back and neck problems)

(a) Place one hand on top of the other on your forehead. Push your head against your hands without moving your head. Hold for a few seconds.

(b) Clasp hands behind head. Push your head back against your hands without moving your head. Hold for a few seconds.

(c) Place right hand on right side of face. Push head against hand without moving. Hold for a few seconds. Repeat other side.

(d) Gently bend head side to side.

(e) Gently turn head from side to side.

(f) Gently bend head forward and backward.

(g) Shrug shoulders up to ears. Breathe in as you shrug your shoulders and out as you relax your shoulders.

(h) Clasp hands, tuck chin in, stretch arms forward as far as you can.

(i) Clasp hands and stretch arms over head.

(j) Clasp hands behind back and stretch.

APPENDIX **III**

Patient Materials (An Example)*

Supportive written material for patients was prepared for Session #1, in which the orientation of the approach is explained in a straightforward and accessible manner. Similar handouts can be developed by the therapist from the material discussed in Chapters 5 through 12, or can be ordered from the publishers.

SESSION 1: CHRONIC PAIN AND THE SELF-MANAGEMENT APPROACH

Orientation

I'd like to start off today by explaining to you the rationale of the self-management approach, which has been found to be the best way to help people with chronic pain problems. I will also explain what is involved in the training, and why you have been selected for a group treatment.

---

*A detailed *Manual for Patients* is now available as a separate publication prepared by Springer Publishing Company, 536 Broadway, New York, NY, 10012, Tel. 212-431-4370.

You are all here because of pain problems (e.g., headache, facial pain, or back pain) that have persisted for some length of time and for which you have been unable to find relief. For many of you, the problem has been becoming worse over the years. Although thoroughly investigated by various specialists, no adequate answer has been found from a physical point of view.

During this time, the view that has been taken of your pain has been very similar to that taken of any injury or acute pain (e.g., when you sprain your ankle or cut your hand). The clinicians have looked for signs of physical damage, or weakness, in your body that can be associated with the pain you are experiencing.

As you probably know, when you injure your body tissue, messages travel with great speed from the injury up to the brain (see Figure AIII.1). The messages are then interpreted, or decoded, by your brain (just like a computer's action) and you become conscious of discomfort . . . you hurt . . . you feel pain.

The discomfort and suffering has an important function. It leads you to:

- remove your body from further damage or danger;
- seek a protected place to rest; and
- eliminate or reduce your usual activities or involvements.

All these actions allow the tissue to heal. Once it has healed and no longer hurts when you use it or move it, and when you can *see* the injury is healed (scar tissue formed, swelling reduced, etc.), you return gradually to your normal activities. The amount you suffer is closely related to the amount your body has been injured.

Experts now realize that this is much too simple an approach to pain. Although of some use in acute pain, it makes less and less sense when one considers chronic or persistent pain problems.

If your pain problem began with an injury to the back or face, that damage healed in approximately six weeks. *And yet the pain persisted.* If your pain has developed without an external injury (e.g., chest pain, headache, jaw pain), there has not been any tissue damage, *and yet pain persists.*

In either case the useful tactic of rest and reduction of your usual routine brings little, if any, relief and may even be producing more severe pain. WHY?

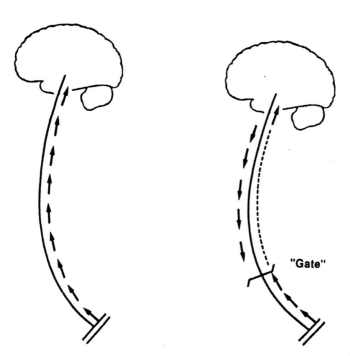

FIGURE AIII(1) Traditional view of pain, as a consequence of, for example, injury to the leg.

FIGURE AIII(2) Contemporary view of pain, as a consequence of, for example, injury to the leg.

Messages coming to the brain from your muscles, skin, ligaments, and internal organs are only *one* ingredient in determining how much you suffer. It is necessary to include a number of other factors that are important influences on pain experience. These influences become increasingly important as pain continues *after healing*, or when pain occurs in repeated episodes of distress (e.g., in headache without any apparent physical injury).

The messages running up to your brain are modulated or affected by messages that come *down* from your brain. These result in the intensity of the nerve impulse being changed or even blocked. Scientists now view pain as a mechanism (rather like a gate) that can influence how much of the nerve messages continue to the brain for interpretation [see Figure AIII (2)].

Let me give you some examples that will illustrate this "gate" in operation.

1. Soccer Injury: If your leg is injured in a soccer game as you battle to retain your one goal lead, you may fail to notice the cut you sustained.
2. Battle Injury: In studies of soldiers wounded in World War II, it was found that many of them felt little pain on the battlefield, and when safely in the hospital they asked for fewer pain killers than civilian patients recovering from operations.
3. If your finger is crushed in a car door, the pain you experience, and the actions you take afterward, will be affected by the situations you are in:
    (a) en route to pick up your lottery winnings;
    (b) en route to the dentist for a root canal;
    (c) while looking after your child, who is severely ill.
4. Hypnosis: In certain types of people, pain can be affected, for short periods of time, by hypnosis—a mode of treatment that operates on one's mental state.
5. In bed at night with no distractions, many of you will have noticed how intense and unbearable the pain feels. You have no distractions in that dark, quiet time, and in addition to the potent effect of focus of attention, you are probably low in mood, feeling helpless and defeated, a state of mind that makes pain more intense.

It is clear from one's own experience, now confirmed by scientists, that pain is affected by many factors and not just the extent of an injury. Experts have now identified a range of factors that influence the amount a person suffers. Put another way, they have clarified the factors that influence the position of that "gate" and consequently the amount of stimulation reaching the brain for interpretation.

The types of factors that are now known to make pain worse are as follows:

1. *Physical Factors*
    (a) Extent of injury and/or degenerative changes.

(b) Extent of residual scarring and other physical reactions to the original injury after healing (e.g., ischemic conditions, fibromyocitis inflammations, and other soft tissue changes).

(c) Nonspecific changes (e.g., in bite symmetry, mild spinal stenosis).

(d) Malfunctioning of artery or muscle system, probably due to an inherited weakness.

(e) Muscle tension.

Many minor physical changes can contribute to pain levels, even though they do not all show up on an x-ray, have been found to be nonprogressive, and imply no necessary physical intervention.

2. *Emotional Factors*
   (a) Anxiety, worry, tension.
   (b) Anger and high levels of excitement.
   (c) Depression.

These factors may be provoked by pain itself or by other life stresses.

3. *Mental Factors*
   (a) Degree of focusing upon the pain.
   (b) Boredom (often resulting from reducing activities to combat pain itself).
   (c) Beliefs and attitudes about the meaning of the pain (e.g., compare the intensity of chest pain believed due to indigestion with that believed to be a precursor of a heart attack). "The pain is a sign of a catastrophic illness or injury."
   (d) Lack of control over pain (e.g., lowered pain tolerance). Many chronic pain sufferers feel no control. "Pain rules my life," is a common theme. "I am helpless to deal with the pain."

However, by the same thinking, it has become evident to experts that the pain can be reduced by similar types of factors. The "gate" can be shifted so as to reduce, if not prevent, the nerve impulses from moving up to the brain and thus reduce pain intensity.

Factors found to reduce pain levels include the following:

1. *Physical Factors*
   These are the major means currently used by doctors to help their patients reduce pain.
   (a) Drugs (sedatives, antiinflammatories, analgesics, etc.).
   (b) Counterstimulation (heat, massage, acupuncture).
   (c) Surgery (e.g., to sever the nerve fiber or fuse vertebrae, etc.).
   (d) Reduced muscular tension and arousal.
2. *Emotional Factors*
   (a) Relaxation and calm.
   (b) Reduced anxiety and, where possible, increased optimism or pleasure (reduced depression).
   (c) Isolation or rest.
3. *Mental Factors*
   (a) Distractions (intense concentration).
   (b) External focus of attention (i.e., on your environment, outside your body).
   (c) Attitude of active coping and control over pain.
   (d) More realistic interpretation of the significance of the pain—no catastrophizing.

All of you are able to identify some of these influences on *your* suffering, though there are, of course, individual differences. Some of you may find one factor much more relevant and potent than others. The interplay among the factors I have been discussing is complex and varies among persons. It is for this reason that we use a "smorgasbord" approach to pain management, providing you with a number of techniques to control pain and asking you to try each one and decide which is most useful for your problem. It is to be hoped that, as our knowledge grows, we will be able to predict better which are the most effective techniques for a particular person.

Some of these factors affecting your pain, however, have proved to be effective only for acute injury and are inadequate when used with chronic problems. I shall be discussing each in more detail later. But, just for a moment, consider the effects of:

1. Drugs: Addiction, side-effects (poor concentration, dizziness, fatigue), tolerance, and even pain exacerbation with prolonged use.
2. Rest/inactivity: Although a useful and natural impulse in acute injury, in chronic pain it can lead to boredom, depression, and muscular atrophy, as well as weakness, loneliness, and preoccupation with unpleasant sensations. All of these reactions make pain feel more severe. A strategy that is useful in promoting healing in acute injury may serve to make pain worse once healing is complete.
3. Surgery: Can lead to new physical problems: scar tissue; soreness; and, in some cases, the pain continues or increases.

It is important to understand that the pain you feel is not merely a function of physical changes. It is also dramatically influenced by emotional and mental factors that can be exploited in your favor; you can learn to modify and manage pain so that you control the amount of pain you experience. The physical "cause" you have been seeking—though a sensible first step with acute injury—is only a preliminary one in dealing with chronic pain. As pain persists, other factors become increasingly important in influencing the pain. A number of vicious cycles can develop that result in making your pain worse. The treatment program provides you with a means of learning to control and manage your own pain.

You may feel that some of the experts you have consulted have implied that, because they cannot remove or relieve your pain by physical methods, it is "in your mind." This can appear to deny the validity of your experience, and relocate the pain in your head, or in your imagination. If you look again at Figure AIII(2), p. 225, and think about this more accurate account of chronic pain, you will realize that *all pain* is "in the mind" (i.e., interpreted as pain by your brain!).

The messages go up to the brain, where the interpretation or perception occurs. This is true whether you have just cut your finger or have continuous backache. With chronic pain, however, the emotional and mental reactions to pain may begin to make it worse. The way you cope with the pain may produce more problems or act to further "open the gate."

The idea that pain which is not closely related to an identifiable injury or illness is "imaginary" is based on the traditional model [Figure AIII(1)].

Let me be more precise about how our own reactions to continuing pain can make the pain worse. When you hurt yourself, your continuing pain leads you to withdraw and rest in order to aid recuperation. But in your cases, rather than recovering, you seem to get worse. The isolation leads you to get bored and depressed. Your physical endurance and fitness decrease. You become fatigued more easily, straining muscles when you expect them to work for you as usual. In one week of total immobility, a muscle will lose one-third of its size and power. If you have seen someone's arm or leg after a cast is removed, you will recall how thin and weak it looked.

Alone and undistracted, pain is more intense; you focus on it, and that, in itself, affects your tolerance of it.

You take drugs to reduce your suffering and they become addictive and produce side-effects (e.g., unclear thinking, drowsiness, gastric difficulties, etc.). In addition, they gradually work less and less efficiently. The drugs may inhibit, or stop, your own production of a natural morphine-like substance that otherwise would help reduce your awareness of pain. In this situation, you become anxious about the pain and your situation, and tense your muscles. You become depressed, unwilling and unmotivated to become active, and bewildered as to what to do. This can lead you to feel helpless and defeated.

Now, looking back at the list of factors that make pain worse, you will see that nearly all of them have arisen as a *consequence* of your reaction to prolonged pain. A set of at least three interlinked vicious cycles emerge [Figure AIII(3)].

In light of these vicious cycles we have developed methods of managing pain that are specifically designed to:

1. Break these cycles.
2. Teach you alternative ways of dealing with pain that help "close the gate" and reduce the sensations, anxiety, and depression, so that you gain understanding and control over this problem by *your own actions.*
3. Encourage you to adopt a different way of living that keeps you well and able to use these methods.

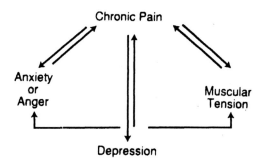

FIGURE AIII(3) Vicious cycles.

The method is called *self-management of chronic pain*. The method consists of:

1. Nine 1 1/2-hour sessions in consecutive weeks to teach you the self-management skills you will need.
2. Daily homework assignments in practicing the skills being taught at sessions.
3. Graded reduction of medication, as your treatment progresses and you learn alternative ways to control the pain.
4. Graded increase in daily activity and specific exercises designed to suit your own needs and strengths and to tone your muscles.

WHAT CAN YOU EXPECT?

For many of you, the problems you have are not new; they have been dragging on for many years.

The self-management approach will lead to a *gradual* and steady improvement, but not to sudden miracles. It will need your active work outside the sessions here with me, practicing coping skills and moving toward an approach to your problem that is directed and controlled by you. When you finish your two months of work, you will have made a significant start and will continue improving afterwards. I would like you to see these sessions as the beginning of a new way of dealing with your problem—slow and gradual, but persistent. As long as you are progressing, even if your pace is slow, you will reach your goal!

It is the general approach found to be most useful and is now used, with some differences, in pain centers all over the country. It leads to approximately 80% of patients improving, increasing their capacity to participate in and enjoy their lives, ceasing to use drugs and reducing their depression.

WHY ARE YOU BEING SEEN IN A GROUP?

1. Although there are differences among you in the locations of your pain and your particular reactions, some common features are prominent.
   (a) Mood change: depression, anxiety, frustration (help-lessness).
   (b) Muscular reaction to pain (or other stresses) in head, neck, and back (muscle tension and spasms; muscle weak-nesses).
   (c) Social withdrawal or overcommitment.
   (d) Reduction in physical and general activities; in a minority of chronic pain sufferers, these social and physical with-drawals are occurring between excessive activity/strain, halted only by pain episodes. Sometimes people report that originally they responded with excessive activity, but over time they gave up and ended up being inactive.
2. People are better motivated to change if they have the support and encouragement of a group whose members are also combating the same problem. Other members of the group understand how it feels.
3. The same techniques are relevant (with some minor adjustments) for all of you, and it is therefore cost-effective to teach, explain, and demonstrate to a group. This cuts down your time for treat-ment, a factor of relevance to each of you.

APPENDIX IV

Therapist Aids for Group Treatment Sessions

These are useful aids for the therapist when working with groups. They allow you to summarize information about the group and keep each patient's problems in mind. In addition, there are sheets [Figures AIV(1) and AIV(2)] to help the therapist keep account of each person's response to the homework assignments and tactics being taught.

GROUP SUMMARY SHEET

Onset Date: _March_

Name	Age	Problem	Chronicity	Average Intensity (0 - 5)	C vs E*	Medication Use	Pre-treatment exercise level and capacity	Other relevant issues (sleep problems, employment issues, relationship difficulties, etc)
Celia Gaites	33	Low back pain	10 yr	3.5	C	Av. of 8 Fraset 292	nil	- hurakwally pain 5/7 nights - adisis avoidance - extensive leg time resting - anxiety abouts re pain + future issue

FIGURE AIV(1) Group summary sheet to be prepared by therapist before beginning group in order to clarify needs, problems, and characteristics of the group.

*Continuous versus episodic.

NAME	Carly Smith
Pre-treatment evalua-tion of goal sheets	✓
Exercise monitoring	✓
Regular exercise	✓✓✓✓
Self-monitoring	-✓✓✓✓
Diaphragmatic breathing	✓✓✓✓ ✓✓✓
Relaxation practice	✓✓✓✓ ✓✓✓
Medication reduction	✓✓✓✓ ✓✓✓
Stress monitoring	✓
Defusing stresses	✓
Distraction techniques	✓
Assertion techniques	unwilling to try
Reappraisal techniques	✓
Self-talk techniques	min. Motive
Activity pacing	✓
Cue-controlled relaxation	✓
Non-avoidance	✓
Strategy comparison	✓

FIGURE AIV(2) Example of a group participation sheet. Check for each individual in group, if and when they complete the homework assignment. Items 3 through 7 can be checked off at each of the 9 sessions.

APPENDIX V

Structured Interview

The structured interview, developed for screening patients and identifying any concomitant problems that they may have, takes approximately one and a half hours to complete and needs to be used in conjunction with questionnaires such as those itemized in Appendix VI. It is not possible for patients to provide all of the information unaided, and it provides a structure for the interview (see the Chronic Pain Assessment Interview Outline). Some sections can be extracted and given to patients to undertake prior to seeing the therapist (estimation of consequences, ameliorators and exacerbators, associated symptoms). However, if the time can be given by the psychologist, he or she will find it useful to personally ask these questions. In answering the interview questions, for example on *consequences*, many details on incapacity, or lack of incapacity, can be collected. In discussing sleep disorders, the patient may initially describe a sleep loss of a certain percentage, but on questioning, it will become evident that he or she has a lifelong history of insomnia or has been subject to early morning awakening since a mood deterioration. A person who describes him or herself as 90% incapacitated in ability to perform physical exercise may go on to reveal that he or she has never done any exercise and had been unfit long before the onset of the pain problem.

CHRONIC PAIN ASSESSMENT INTERVIEW OUTLINE

Date: _____ Hospital Number: _____
Name: _____
Referral source: _____
Referral date: _____
Reason for referral: _____
Address: _____

Marital status: _____
Currently living with (relationship): _____
Occupation: _____
Present working status: _____
Qualifications/education (max): _____

Presenting Problem

_____

_____
_____
_____
_____
_____

Average pain symptoms (from self-monitoring diaries, when possible)
(1) Rated average intensity (0–5): _____
(2) Peak intensity (0–5): _____
(3) Frequency per week/month: _____
(4) Duration (average hours): _____
(5) Onset focus and laterality: _____
(6) Spread: _____
(7) Patterning of episodes: _____
     Course: static, gradually worsening, sudden worsening, gradual improvement,
     fluctuating, other: _____
(8) Accompanying symptoms:

Vomiting	_____	Numbness/tingling	_____
Nausea	_____	Heart beating fast	_____
Dizziness	_____	Heart beating loud	_____
Feeling faint	_____	Noise sensitivity	_____
Fear	_____	Light sensitivity	_____
Rapid breathing	_____	Irritability	_____
Sweating	_____	Palpitations	_____
Blurred vision	_____	Anxiety	_____
Visual prodroma	_____	Depression	_____

Others _____

Antecedents/exacerbators/ameliorators of symptom
(Mark – if exacerbator; + if ameliorator; * if considered a trigger of episode)
 1. Worry: _____
 2. Tension: _____
 3. Physical exercise, movement (standing, lifting, walking, etc.): _____
 4. Menstrual cycle: _____
 5. Relaxation: _____
 6. Weekends: _____
 7. Vacations: _____
 8. Going to work: _____
 9. Concentration: _____
10. Reading: _____
11. Studying: _____
12. Listening to lectures, seminars, talks, etc.: _____
13. Noises: _____
14. Excitement: _____
15. Quarrels: _____
16. Anger: _____
17. Emotional times: _____
18. Sunshine: _____
19. Hot baths: _____
20. Precision work: _____
21. Sex: _____
22. Annoyances: _____
23. Diet—certain food and/or drink: _____
24. Alcohol: _____
25. Fatigue: _____
26. Weather: _____
27. Sympathy & attention: _____
28. Cold/heat: _____
29. Others: _____

Consequences: Since the onset of your problem, has your participation in the following changed? (estimate % interference of pain in:)

		Description
Physical exercise	_____%	_____
Activities	_____%	_____
Leisure/social	_____%	_____
Sexual activity	_____%	_____
Daily life	_____%	_____
Sleeping	_____%	_____
Relationships	_____%	_____
Housework & chores	_____%	_____

Daily routine

_____

_____

_____

_____

Past and present medication use

Name	Time on Medication	Dose	Time/Day	Effectiveness and/or Reason for Discontinuing
_____	_____	_____	_____	_____
_____	_____	_____	_____	_____
_____	_____	_____	_____	_____

Interviewer's assessment of patient's attitudes to use and dependence:

_____

Average number of cigarettes per day: _____

Average tea/coffee intake per day: _____

Use of contraceptive pill: Yes _____ No _____

Use of other psychoactive drugs (cocaine, marijuana, amphetamines, etc.):

Alcohol (frequency/amount): current: _____

past: _____

Coping strategies (excluding avoidance):

	Type	% of time used to control pain	Effectiveness (0–10)
1.	_____	_____	_____
2.	_____	_____	_____
3.	_____	_____	_____
4.	_____	_____	_____
5.	_____	_____	_____
6.	_____	_____	_____
7.	_____	_____	_____
8.	_____	_____	_____
9.	_____	_____	_____
10.	_____	_____	_____

History of current problem

_____

_____

_____

_____

_____

_____

_____

Previous treatments/specialist consultations & outcome
(date, type, efficacy, attitude to, etc.):
1. _____

2. _____

3. _____

4. _____

_____

Hospitalizations/operations:
1. _____
2. _____
3. _____
4. _____
Outcome: _____

_____

General
Physical health—general (other somatic problems):
_____

_____

_____

Family:
Relationships: _____

_____

History of psychiatric problems: _____

_____

History of pain/disability: _____

_____

History of abuse, neglect: _____

_____

Attitudes to pain/illness: _____

_____

_____

Childhood: (quality, siblings, health, social, etc.):

_____

_____

_____

_____

_____

Marital history:

Age at marriage: _____ Age of spouse: _____

Occupation of spouse: _____ Working now? _____

Length of marriage: _____

Other marriages: _____

Number of children: _____ Ages: _____

Description of marriage: _____

_____

Major causes of conflict: (financial, children, parents, in-laws, work, personality differences, sexual problems, physical illness, religion, other: _____

_____

How do people you live with know you are in pain? _____

_____

_____

Reaction of family/spouse, etc. to pain episodes and disabilities:

     encourage/supportive   _____

     ignore/angry   _____

     distract   _____

     encourage to be active despite   _____

     encourage to avoid   _____

Psychiatric history and current problems:

Depression: sad mood, insomnia/hypersomnia or sleep difficulties, suicide thoughts, lack of appetite, weight gain or loss (_____ lbs), loss of interest, guilt, fatigue, diurnal fluctuations, loss of sexual interest, poor concentration, irritability, anhedonic. _____

     Past history of: _____

_____

Anxiety: tension, tremor, physical manifestations, pain, phobias. _____

_____

     Past history of: _____

_____

Impression of personality: _____

Evidence of: obsessional/compulsive problems, eating difficulties, hypochondriacal concerns, intellectual impairment, psychotic symptoms, other

_____

_____

Recent and ongoing stresses:

Type	Approximate date of onset	Reaction	Association with pain
_____	_____	_____	_____
_____	_____	_____	_____
_____	_____	_____	_____

Work history
Education: _____

Work history: _____

_____

_____

_____

Present employment (F/PT)
1. Financial situation: _____

2. Work satisfaction: _____

3. Amount of time lost due to pain (in last six months): _____

4. Problems with job: _____

If currently not working:
1. Means of support: _____

2. Job availability and need of retraining: _____

3. Motivation to return/begin: _____

4. Former working income: _____
   Current benefits (type, size): _____
5. Duration of compensation: _____
6. Stage of current or planned litigation: _____

7. Satisfaction with current status: _____

Patient's view of problem and its cause(s) and likely course:
_____
_____

If pain disappeared, what would you wish to do? _____
_____

Outlook for future: _____
_____

Expectations of clinic: _____
_____

Behavior during interview: _____
_____

SUMMARY SHEET

Evidence of:

1. Depression: _____

2. Anxiety: _____

3. Avoidance/confrontation activity patterns: _____
   _____

4. Inactivity/unfit: _____

5. No evolved coping strategies: _____

6. Drug dependency: _____

7. Poor/inadequate understanding of chronic pain/physical mechanicisms: _____
   _____

8. Work disruption: _____

9. Marital problems: _____

10. Other: _____
    _____

11. Motivation for self-management: _____

12. Sources of secondary gain:
    (a) financial
    (b) sympathy, attention, support from significant others and health care workers
    (c) provision of time to engage in preferred activities
    (d) avoidance of work, school, unpleasant duties (e.g., home or family related), social events
    (e) other

13. Cognitions:
    What does the pain signify for the patient?
    How does the patient view the pain?
    How modifiable is it?
    How hopeful are they about improvement?
    How realistic is their assessment of the problem?
    How passive or active can they be in modifying the pain?

14. Supplementary testing:
    Behavioral tests, cognitive tests, McGill Pain Index, tests of depression/anxiety

APPENDIX **VI**

Measurement Instruments

These measuring instruments have been found useful in a chronic pain assessment service that utilizes the approach described in this manual. References to articles on each of the questionnaires on the following pages are provided in the suggested readings at the end of Chapter 3. With the rapid growth of research into the nature and assessment of pain, new instruments appear with regularity. The present selection of tests should be useful, but is not exhaustive.

COGNITIONS

In a study of 127 patients with chronic pains of various types (Philips, 1987b), the heterogeneity of the cognitions was apparent from the emergence of several clusters of cognitions, including thoughts about social withdrawal, frustration and disappointment with oneself, feelings of helplessness, concern of the affects of the pain, and expressions of emotional reactivity to the pain. The positive cognitions concerned coping, and the most important of these items, which explained 18% of the variance, were: reassuring thoughts that one can cope because one has coped in the past, deliberate use of distraction techniques, reminding oneself to be optimistic, and accepting the pain to an extent. A complete list of these cognitions reported by patients as common whenever they experienced the onset of a severe episode of pain is given in the following pages.

As described in Chapter 13, the most common negative-cognition factors are: helplessness, uncontrollability, catastrophizing.

The following list of references contains a selection of recent studies on cognitive measurement.

SUGGESTED READINGS

Brown, G. K., & Nicassio, P. M. (1987). Development of a questionnaire for the assessment of active and passive coping strategies in chronic pain patients. *Pain, 31*(1), 53–64.

Flor, H., & Behle, D. J. (1993). Assessment of pain related cognitions in chronic pain patients. *Behavior Research and Therapy, 31*(1), 63–73.

Flor, H., & Turk, D. C. (1988). Chronic back pain and rheumatoid arthritis: Predicting pain and disability from cognitive variables. *Journal of Behavioral Medicine, 11*(3), 251–265.

Lefebvre, M. F. (1981). Cognitive distortion and cognitive errors in depressed psychiatric and low back pain patients. *Journal of Consulting and Clinical Psychology, 49*(4), 517–525.

Melzack, R. (Ed.). (1983). *Pain measurement and assessment.* New York: Raven Press.

Philips, H. C. (1989). Thoughts provoked by pain. *Behavior Research and Therapy, 27*(4), 469–473.

Pilowsky, I., & Katsikitis, M. (1994). A classification of illness behavior in pain clinic patients. *Pain, 57,* 91–94.

Rosenstiel, A. K., & Keefe, F. J. (1983). The use of coping strategies in chronic low back pain patients: Relationship to patient characteristics and current adjustment. *Pain, 17*(1), 33–44.

Smith, T., & Peck, J. (1988). Cognitive distortion in rheumatoid arthritis: Relation to depression and disability. *Journal of Consulting and Clinical Psychology, 56,* 412–416.

Williams, D. A., & Thorn, B. E. (1989). An empirical assessment of pain beliefs. *Pain, 36*(3), 351–358.

THE MCGILL PAIN QUESTIONNAIRE

Description	Interpretation
A 78-descriptor scale arranged in 20 subscales that is used to measure pain experience. It can be scored in order to give measures of both intensity and quality of pain experience and has been shown to have three components: sensory, affective, and evaluative	Philips & Jahanshahi, 1985, have provided the following norms on chronic headache from a sample of 352 patients with at least a 1-year history: —NWC $= 11.1\ (4.4)$ —PRIS $= 15.9\ (7.9)$ —PRIA $=\ 4.9\ (3.3)$ —PRIE $=\ 3.5\ (1.7)$ [Shaughnessy Back Pain Clinic ($n = 134$) unpublished] —NWC $= 12.37\ (4.03)$ —PRIS $= 13.18\ (7.15)$ —PRIA $=\ 4.07\ (4.3)$ —PRIE $=\ 3.2\ (2.0)$

[Melzack, R. (1975). The McGill Pain Questionnaire: Major properties and scoring methods. *Pain, 1,* 277–299]

PAIN BEHAVIOR QUESTIONNAIRE

Description	Interpretation
A 38-item inventory of behavior (pp. 250–251) in which individuals can tick the presence or absence of a behavior in their behavioral repertoire (in response to pain). Six distinguishable types of avoidance behavior have been found to account for 42.6% of the total variance. Two factors of complaint (verbal and non-verbal) are distinguishable.	Each factor can be analyzed separately &/or a total avoidance and complaint factor derived. In a chronic headache sample ($n = 267$). —mean total avoidance $= 17.7(7.9)$ —total complaint $= 2.62\ (1.3)$

Philips, H. C., & Jahanshahi, M. (1985). The components of pain behavior report. *Behavior Research & Therapy, 24*(2), 117–125

BEHAVIORAL RESPONSES TO PAIN

When you have an episode of pain, what is your usual response? Make a mark
anywhere on the lines from ''Not at all'' to ''Always.''

Not at all   Usually   Always

1. Avoid lifting objects
2. Lie down/rest/sleep
3. Grimace, frown, pull face
4. Avoid restaurants
5. Tell friend
6. Have alcohol
7. Avoid gardening
8. Take prescribed medication
9. Cry
10. Avoid party-going
11. Avoid housework
12. Avoid public transportation
13. Have massage
14. Avoid standing
15. Avoid going to work
16. Sign, moan, cry out
17. Tell someone in family
18. Go swimming
19. Apply heat
20. Take unprescribed medication
21. Avoid movie theatres
22. Avoid travel in cars
23. Avoid shopping
24. Change posture
25. Avoid cleaning car
26. Avoid walking
27. Avoid bright lights
28. Avoid sex

29. Avoid having visitors
30. Avoid odd jobs in house
31. Slow down in physical movements
32. Avoid carrying
33. Avoid loud noise
34. Rub, stroke site of pain
35. Avoid visiting
36. Avoid cooking
37. Avoid bending
38. Avoid walking stairs

COGNITIVE EVALUATION SCALE

Description	Interpretation
A 48-item scale that includes thoughts and feelings that individuals may notice at the onset of the pain episode or when pain intensifies. Subjects indicate how representative the responses are to their reaction to pain using a 0–3 scale.	Penzien et al. (1985), using it for headache only, has provided results indicative of the presence of a number of separable factors, or types of cognitions association with pain. Philips (1987c) evaluated the factorial structure of cognitions of a large sample of chronic pain sufferers using a modification of this scale. The following norms may be of use: Mean = 52.6 (22.4) [Shaughnessy Back Pain Clinic (n = 134) unpublished]

[Pensien et al. (1985). *Journal of Psychosomatic Res. 27*(5), 431–440]
[Bakal, D. A. (1982). *Psychobiology of chronic headache.* New York: Springer Publishing Co. (p. 135)]

STATE-TRAIT ANXIETY INVENTORY

Description	Interpretation
Two 20-item inventories that assess anxiety traits (trait and state). Each item is answered on a scale from 0 to 4 to indicate intensity. Norms are provided by the author for university students, neurological psychiatric patients, general medical patients, as well as prisoners.	Norms allow raw scores to be converted to percentile ranks for state and trait scores against appropriate groups.

[Spielberger et al. (1970). *Manual for the STAI.* Palo Alto, CA: Consulting Psychologist's Press.]

SICKNESS IMPACT PROFILE

Description	Interpretation
A 136-item self-report measure yielding 12 subscale scores reflecting a range of areas in which dysfunctional behavior may be present. Overall impairment scores are calculated, as well as summary scores of physical and psychosocial dysfunction.	Possible range of scores is from 0 to 100%. Average overall score in the general population is estimated to be 3.6. In chronic low back pain patients average score would be 23.8, and in rheumatoid arthritic patients, 15.6.

[Bergner et al. (1981). The Sickness Impact Profile: Development and final revision of the health status measure. *Medical Care, 19*, 787–805]

THE BECK DEPRESSION INVENTORY

Description	Interpretation
A 21-item self-report measure yielding numerical estimates of depression and its severity. Patients select one of four (or five) statements, each ranked in order of severity.	Scores range from 0 to 63 0– 9 none 10–14 borderline 15–20 mild 21–30 moderate 31–40 severe 41–63 very severe

[Beck et al. (1961). An inventory of measuring depression. *Archives of General Psychiatry, 4*, 53–63.]

APPENDIX VII

Specific Information Relevant to Headache Management

PHYSIOLOGICAL MECHANISMS

For the most part, this treatment program is useful for all types of chronic pain, and no specific attention need be paid to pain with a particular locus. An exception occurs with severe headache, where the therapist's knowledge of some of the physiological mechanisms involved in vascular headache problems is useful.

Severe headache sufferers are often bewildered by their own symptoms, especially with respect to what are sometimes called "rebound headaches." A clear explanation of the presumed inherited weakness in the stability of the intra- and extracranial arteries in response to stimulation proves a useful model for them to have and one that is easily explained.

There is some controversy about the physiological underpinnings of tension and migraine headache, as well as controversy about the utility of classifying them into two separate groups. There is symptomatic and physiological evidence to suggest a large overlap between the two types of headache, and it is probable that as headaches become more severe they entail more and more vascular concomitants. It is useful for all severe headache sufferers to understand the consequences of instability and variability in cranial arteries and how they may relate to their own pain problems.

The physiological response to arousal and stimulation is a constriction of the cranial arteries followed by a vasodilation, and then a gradual return to normal arterial width. This biphasic response is normal and occurs in all persons under conditions of stimulation. Instability can develop in this response such that prolonged or repeated stress or stimulation leads to overconstriction of the arteries (an overnarrowing of their diameter) and thus to a reduction of the amount of blood that can flow through. In headache-prone people, this overconstriction is the explanation of the curious symptoms that are experienced prior to the onset of pain (visual effects, smells, feelings, gastric sensations, and even numbness in the fingers and toes or extreme coldness of the hands). This is followed by an overdilation of the artery in the body's attempt to return the cranial arteries back to a normal state (homeostasis). During this overdilating period, patients can experience severe pain and sometimes vomiting. They may feel a flushing and heat in their face in association with the pounding and intense pain.

Sufferers from migraine have inherited an instability in this arterial activity and appear more prone to overconstriction and the resultant overdilation. This biphasic pattern, in its extreme form, is the one they are tussling with and the one that needs to be normalized in their attempts to manage headache. Explaining this pattern will allow them to gain a better understanding of why they so often are struck down with severe pain when they relax on the weekends, at the beginning of vacations, and perhaps even when they awake in the morning. In response to relaxation and the cessation of stimulation, the cranial arterial system is thrown into a rebound response that leads to an overdilation and severe pain.

Understanding the symptomatology in this way allows migraine patients to begin to think of activity pacing and the need for relaxation techniques in a specific way. Their goal is to prevent overdilation or, more positively, to increase the stability of the temporal arteries by reducing persistent overstimulation or repeated activation. Preventing long periods or extreme periods of constriction makes rebound less likely. Slowing down gradually after a period of intense stress or activity, allowing themselves periods of relaxation between intense demand, and reducing the demands made on themselves where possible are all strategies that are worth considering for them.

In addition, the effects of certain foods, drinks, menstrual cycle, and drugs can be better explained with this model of inherited arterial instability. The goal of reducing the instability by control of effector variables becomes a tangible and appropriate challenge with a realistic base. Even under perfect conditions, patients may have some migraines, but many can be reduced, aborted, or eliminated.

FOOD SENSITIVITIES

Tyramine, a chemical that is thought to dilate blood vessels, has sufficiently high concentrations in some foods to make a contribution to the food sensitivities some migraine sufferers have reported. There are certain cheeses that are particularly high in tyramine: mature cheeses like stilton, brie, emmenthaler, and camembert. Chocolate has long been known to be a provoker, and should be avoided by those wishing to try an exclusionary diet. Citrus fruits have been reported to produce attacks more commonly than other types of fruit, though some people have reported that unripe apples can be troublesome.

Pickled herring and marmite contain very large concentrations of tyramine, while cheese, alcoholic beverages, and chocolate also contain several other amines with an action very similar to that of tyramine. Some people find that they can drink white wine but not red, the latter being the alcohol most often reported to be an exacerbator.

There are no clear-cut diagnostic tests for these types of sensitivities, and the standard skin tests for food allergies often give negative results when patients have these allergies. Although complete exclusionary diets are complex and difficult to undertake, a patient can decide to eliminate certain of the high tyramine foods for a period of time and see if it has any noticeable effect on the control of the pain problem.

There are some people who are extremely sensitive to monosodium glutamate, found in high concentrations in most Chinese cuisine. It can lead to headache, chiefly in the temples and forehead, and is often found in association with feelings of tightness or pressure over the face and chest.

All migraine sufferers should be advised to eat on a regular schedule, and to avoid dramatic slimming diets. During an attack it is important to try to eat and to drink (if only small quantities), especially something that contains carbohydrates, such as starch or sugar, because of the association of lack of food with headache exacerbation. Needless to say, when the headache is so severe that vomiting is occurring, this will be impossible; however, at the early stages of headache it is advisable and may prevent a more severe attack.

In advising patients about how to undertake a check on the effects of a particular food or drink for their headache problems, the therapist should advise them to take one particular food that they are interested in assessing and avoid it for a definite period of time (e.g., one month). If there is no change in the frequency over the full month, then this substance can be reintroduced and the next one experimented with (e.g., cheese for one month, followed by chocolate for one month with the reintroduction of cheese). If headaches are very infrequent, the omission of a certain food will have to go on for longer periods of time in order to provide a proper assessment of the association.

MENSTRUATION AND MIGRAINE

It has long been known that there is a strong association between vascular headaches and the endocrine system. The most common time for headaches for women is before menstruation and, not uncommonly, at the time of ovulation. Often severe headache problems clear up during pregnancy. In addition, contraceptive pills, which modulate endocrine levels, can cause attacks of migraine, probably because of the estrogen content. It is for this reason that patients are advised to discontinue use of their oral contraceptives if they have a severe headache problem *prior* to the onset of treatment. Alternative methods of contraception can be substituted before interrupting use of the oral contraceptive.

The understanding of the vulnerability of a person at certain times of the month is an important piece of information to make available to them, as it helps them in the management of their headaches. The recognition of a vulnerable week well ahead of time allows women to pace their activities and put less demand on themselves during that premenstrual week. In addition, the understanding of the mechanisms that may be operative helps one to appraise the pain appropriately and limit the catastrophic interpretations and anxiety that may occur during episodes.

APPENDIX VIII

Exercise Monitoring Sheets

Figure AVIII(1) is a grid for the daily monitoring of general or specific flexion exercises. The former can be monitored in number of minutes of exercising, while the latter can be monitored in number of cycles of each exercise.

The monitoring sheet will help increase compliance as well as allowing the therapist a quick method of monitoring each participant's exercise work as treatment progresses. Explaining the columns and rows to patients when first giving the sheet to them will save a good deal of confusion later in treatment. The column marked "days" is used to enter the days of the week, beginning on the day after you give out this form. The column marked "assess" refers to their assessment of their own capacity during the first week of monitoring, in which they note down their actual levels of exercise *without adjusting them*. From this can be derived an average level, which it is wise for them to begin in week two. Thus, from week two onward, the therapist is looking for a *gradual* increase in exercise levels and compliance with daily exercise routines. The minimum to be achieved over the nine-week program is 20 to 30 minutes of brisk walking *daily*. Specific exercises can usefully be increased to 10 to 20 times daily. Notice that this sheet allows patients to continue monitoring after the nine-week program ends.

Name: _Celia Gaites_

Treatment Onset Date: _March_

General Fitness: Please indicate the total number of minutes of either swimming/walking/bicycling per day (column) for each week of treatment. Record only consecutive exercise time (not, for example, walking time when shopping, etc.).

OR

Specific Exercises: Please indicate your daily total number of repetitions of exercises (pelvic tilts, sit-ups, etc.) achieved each day (column) for each week of treatment.

Day	Assess	Week												
		2	3	4	5	6	7	8	9	10	11	12	13	14
Tues	0	9	11	13	15	17	18	20	25					
Wed	20	9	11	13	15	17	18	20	25					
Thur	5	9	11	13	15	17	18	20	25					
Fri	0	9	11	13	15	17	18	20	25					
Sat	40	–	11	13	15	–	18	20	25					
Sun	0	9	11	13	15	–	18	20	25					
Mon	0	9	11	–	15	–	18	20	25					

FIGURE AVIII(1)   Example of general exercise and specific exercise monitoring sheet.

APPENDIX IX

Complaint (Verbal/Nonverbal) Monitoring

Name: _Celie Gaites_   Date: _April 6_

Please tick below each time you notice any of the items below during the
next few days, and return to me. Use one row to indicate the frequency of
complaining or discussions of problem for one day (24-hour period) and
mark date.

Date	Complaining of pain and discomfort or handicap	Discussion of problem (or related issues such as medication, doctor's appt., disability due to pain, etc.).
April 6	✔ ✔ ✔ ✔	✔ ✔
7	—	✔
8	✔ ✔ ✔ ✔ ✔ ✔	✔ ✔ ✔
9	✔ ✔	✔ ✔ ✔ ✔
10	✔ ✔ ✔	✔
11	✔	✔ ✔ ✔ ✔ ✔
12	✔ ✔ ✔ ✔ ✔ ✔ ✔	—

FIGURE AIX(1)   Example of patient monitoring sheet of pain complaint and/
or discussion of pain problem.

Observer's Name: ___Joe Gaites___ Date: ___April 6___

Relationship to Patient (e.g., husband, wife, child, close friend, mother, etc.): _____

Please tick below each time you notice any of the items below during the next few days, and return to me. Use one row to indicate the frequency of complaining or discussions of problem for one day (24-hour period) and mark date.

Date	Complaining of pain and discomfort or handicap	Discussion of problem (or related issues such as medication, doctor's appt., disability due to pain, etc.).
6	✓	✓ ✓ ✓
7	✓	✓ ✓ ✓ ✓ ✓ ✓
8	—	✓
9	—	✓ ✓
10	✓	—
11	✓ ✓ ✓ ✓ ✓	✓ ✓ ✓ ✓ ✓ ✓ ✓
12	out all the day ／ ?	

FIGURE AIX(2) Example of observer monitoring sheet of pain complaint and/or discussion of pain problem.

APPENDIX **X**

Short Relaxation Induction

ALTERNATIVE 1

Now I'd like you to start off by tuning in to yourself and seeing how you feel, closing your eyes, settling comfortably down into your chair; kick off your shoes if you want to, and notice for a moment where the tension is in your body. Scan yourself from the very top of your head to the bottom of your feet and see if you are holding tension in any particular part of yourself.

Alter your breathing now, so that you are breathing evenly and steadily. Is your breathing shallow and fast, or is it even and deep? Once you have got this picture of your current state, I want you to deepen your breathing very gradually, taking the air right down to the bottom of your lungs and starting a very even, steady exchange of air. Evenly and steadily, knowing that every time you breathe out, you can relax further and further. Feel your chest warm and relaxed as the air flows out of your lungs.

And as you sit there relaxing and breathing evenly and steadily, I want you to see if you can increase the relaxation in each of the parts of the body as I name them. As I name the part, consciously relax that body part as you breathe out, breathing away the tension and using your cue word or image to help you relax.

For example, if we start off with your legs, and I say "I want you to relax your legs," I want you to say to yourself, "relax," as you breathe out, and breathe away the tension from the very top of your hips right down to your feet. Make sure no tension is being held in any of these muscles.

Make sure that your toes are loose; the legs, the knees, the shins, and your thighs, are heavy and relaxed, breathing away the tension, and as you breathe out say to yourself, "relax; let go," breathing away the tension, or using the soothing image that helps you. Whatever the cue is that you associate with deep relaxation, say it to yourself as you breathe out.

Now think about your arms. Are they as relaxed as they could be? If not, on the next OUT breath, make them heavy and tired, hanging beside you, breathing evenly and steadily. Good. Make sure your shoulders are very heavy. Breathing away the tension.

And now think about your buttocks, your stomach, and your midriff. Make sure you are not holding them all very tight. On the OUT breath, let go all those muscles, breathing evenly and steadily. Letting go of the tension on the OUT breath, so that the middle of your body is heavy and relaxed, and your legs and your arms and your chest are relaxed. As you breathe out, you feel the warmth spreading through your chest, the muscles relaxing further.

And now, think about your shoulders. Are they really relaxed? Could you let them go a little bit further now on the OUT breath. Ease the tension in the shoulders, let them hang, don't necessarily rest them on the arms of the chair, but let them hang loosely so that the weight of the shoulders eases away the tension in your neck, breathing evenly and steadily. And now, think about your neck. Make sure your head is well balanced on your shoulders. Now allow the tension in your shoulders to go, down the neck, across the shoulders, and down the arms. Or perhaps, if you'd rather, let the image flow right down your back, the "water" of the tension just flows away, breathing evenly and steadily. Relaxing the front of your neck, relaxing the back of your neck, and breathing away the tension as you say to yourself, "relax," breathing evenly and steadily.

And now, think about all the muscles in your face; all the little muscles around your eyes, across the bridge of your nose, your temples, and your jaw. Let them all loosen up on the OUT breath, let your jaw open slightly, and your tongue move to the front part of your mouth, relaxing your throat and your mouth, your jaw, all the muscles in your eyes. Imagine your eyebrows slowly moving out toward your ears, smoothing away, and then lengthening the muscles. From the top of your head right to the base of your scalp, let the tension flow away from you over the top of your head, breathing evenly and steadily. Good.

Now as you relax, I want you, on every OUT breath, to use your cue word or image as you relax further and further telling yourself to "relax," "relax," "relax," and enjoying that deep relaxation of the muscles that you can achieve in such a short period of time.

And now turn your mind to a peaceful image, keeping it very clearly in your mind's eye, and holding it there—not allowing any other thought to distract you—breathing evenly and steadily, relaxing further and further. Good. Keep breathing and relaxing, further and further. If other thoughts come to your mind's eye, gently push them to one side. As you sit thinking of your soothing scene, I want you to enjoy that feeling of total relaxation in your mind and your body that you have achieved in such a short period of time.

Now I want you to rouse yourself slowly while I count backwards from five. *Five*: move your fingers and toes. *Four*: move your knees and legs. *Three*: begin to rouse yourself, and as you rouse yourself, you are going to come back and feel refreshed and relaxed as if you have just had a short afternoon nap. *Two*: yawn and stretch, and, *one*: open your eyes.

ALTERNATIVE 2

Now what I'd like you to do, is to walk with me down ten steps to deep relaxation. I want you to imagine, with your eyes closed, as you comfortably settle into your chair . . . imagine yourself standing at the top of a flight of ten steps, and we're going to go down these steps together. At the bottom, you are going to be completely relaxed.

On the first step down, I want you to notice your breathing. Make it as even and steady as you can and remember that on the OUT breath you can increase the relaxation of your body a great deal, and by pacing your breathing, you can calm your whole system down, breathing evenly and steadily. See if you can establish a pattern of breathing on this first step that you can use throughout this stepping.

And let's now go on to our second step down, keeping your breathing even, and on the OUT breath, relax your legs and your arms completely so that they hang like heavy weights, floppy, heavy limbs, almost disassociated from you. Breathing away the tension on every OUT breath, even and steady. Heavy and relaxed. Good. And on the third step down, I want you to think about your buttocks, stomach, and chest. See if you can make them even more relaxed. On each OUT breath letting go of the buttocks, letting go of the stomach and midriff, so that they are completely relaxed and acquiescent. Breathing evenly and steadily. Good.

And now, let's take a fourth step down toward complete relaxation by working on the tension in the neck and shoulders. See if you can relax your shoulders and your neck a little bit further. See if you can use the OUT breath to reduce the tension in the neck and make it flow down the shoulders and the back and out of your body, breathing evenly and steadily. Good.

And now concentrate on the muscles in your jaw and face. And on the next OUT breath, loosen your jaw. Let your jaw hang open and breathe away the tension in the jaw, and the temples, all the muscles around the eyes and forehead, lengthening your eyebrows, smooth away the wrinkles and the lines, and tensions in the muscles, breathing evenly and steadily. Good. Keep on breathing and relaxing.

And on the fifth step down, I want you to relax the top of your head right down your spine. Imagine the tension is flowing like water over the top of your head, down the back of your head, and right down your spine, letting yourself rest comfortably in the chair, letting the chair take all of the weight, breathing evenly and steadily, relaxing further and further.

And on the sixth step down, I want you to unwind any differences between the two sides of your body. Imagine an imaginary line running down between your nose, and right down the center of your body, and see if the two sides of your body are perfectly balanced. If you detect that one side is more tense than the other, on the next OUT breath, concentrate on that body part, reducing it further and further, letting the tension really relax away, make it the same as the good side, relaxing further and further. Good.

And on the seventh step down, I want you to start relaxing your mind, too. Focus your attentions on a soothing, peaceful image, far away from here, and if other thoughts come to your mind, gently push them off to one side, you can deal with them at some other time. Now you want to absorb yourself totally in one single, soothing image. Breathing evenly and steadily. Relaxing further and further. Holding the image in your mind's eye and exploring it. Good.

And on the eighth step down I want you to say to yourself on each OUT breath, some word you associate with deep relaxation such as you are feeling at the moment. It might be "relax," "relax," "soothe," "letting go," or it might be a word that reminds you of that image that is most soothing for you ("the sea," "the sea," "the sky"). This word can evoke for you this beautiful, peaceful, balanced state that you can achieve so quickly for yourself. And on the ninth step down, return to your peaceful image. Hold it in your mind and just enjoy this feeling that you have now, and your body is completely relaxed and balanced. There is nothing you need think about other than your soothing scene.

And finally, you step right down to the bottom of the stairs and you are completely relaxed and peaceful, your body is heavy and tired, and your mind is well-balanced, holding the peaceful image. And when you turn around to come back up the steps, you'll find that you have retained this feeling with you, that you will go on feeling peaceful and alert all day. Peaceful and yet alert. These things are not incompatible. You will feel refreshed, as though you have just had a brief sleep.

And as you walk back up the steps, gradually rousing your body as you go. *Nine*, move your feet and toes. *Eight*, move your fingers a little. *Seven*, stretch out your arms, feel the stretch. *Six*, move your legs, stretch your legs a little bit. *Five*, move your shoulders. *Four*, move your head a little bit. *Three*, open your eyes, yawn. And *two*, *one*, coming back to where you began at the top of the stairs.

APPENDIX **XI**

Comparison of Tactics

FORMS

The following page is a useful sheet to help patients evaluate the effects of the tactics they have learned to reduce pain (see Sessions #8 and #9). Ask them to complete it during the next week. All of the tactics previously discussed are itemized, and these can be reviewed with patients to remind them of the meaning of any they have forgotten. They are asked to rate the efficacy of each tactic for them, on a number of occasions, and to come up with a conclusion about its overall usefulness in the management of their pain problem.

PAIN MANAGEMENT TACTICS

Indicate which techniques are proving useful to you by monitoring this week and indicating effect (✓ = tried tactics; + = reduced pain; – = increased pain; NE = no effect). Draw a final conclusion (in last column) after you have tried each a number of times. Star (*) most favored methods for you.

	Tick no. of times tried & effect +/–/NE	Decision re utility +/–/NE	
Diaphragmatic (deep, regular) breathing	✓+, ✓+, ✓+, ✓+, ✓+, ✓+	+	*
Progressive relaxation	✓+, ✓+, ✓NE, ✓+, ✓+, ✓+	+	*
Short relaxation induction ("cue relaxation")	✓+, ✓–, ✓+, ✓+, ✓+	+	
Peaceful imagery	✓+, ✓+, ✓+	+	
External focusing (sounds, stimuli outside body, activity engaged in)	✓+, ✓–, ✓+, ✓+	+	
Mental distraction (thoughts, memories, mathematics . . .)	✓+, ✓– ✓–, ✓+	+/– ?	
Reappraisal (i) transformation of pain	✓–, ✓–, ✓–	–	
(ii) transformation of context or situation	✓–, ✓–	–	
(iii) redefinition of pain	✓+, ✓+, ✓+	+	
(iv) denial of pain	✓–, ✓–	–	
(v) limiting pain	✓–	–	
(vi) relocating pain	✓+, ✓+, ✓+, ✓+	+	*
(vii) relocating your thoughts to a nonpain site	✓+, ✓–, ✓–	–	
Self-talk or Self-statements	✓+, ✓+, ✓+	+	
Persistence or nonavoidance	✓+, ✓–, ✓+	+	
Activity pacing	✓+, ✓+, ✓+, ✓+	+	*
Anxiety reduction/defusing	✓+, ✓+, ✓+, ✓+, ✓+, ✓+	+	**
Exercise	✓+ (daily)	+	*
Direct statement of needs/assertion	✓+, ✓+	+	
Drugs	No longer in use!		
Others: 1. _____			
2. _____			
3. _____			

REFERENCES

(This reference list includes suggested readings from each chapter, cited references, as well as articles or books that have been used as reference notes.)

Abram, S. E., Anderson, R. A., & Maitra deCruze, A. M. (1981). Factors predicting short-term outcomes of nerve blocks in the management of chronic pain. *Pain, 10,* 323–330.

Alberti, R., & Emmons, M. (1982). *Your perfect right.* San Luis Obispo, CA: Impact Publishing.

Alloy, L., & Tabachnik, N. (1984). Assessment of covariation by humans and animals: The joint influence of prior expectations and current situational information. *Psychological Review, 91,* 112–149.

American Psychiatric Association. (1994). *Diagnostic and statistical manual of mental disorders IV (4th Ed.).* Washington, DC: Author.

Arntz, A., & Peters, M. (1995). Chronic low back pain and inaccurate predictions of pain: Is being too tough a risk factor for the development and maintenance of chronic pain? *Behavior Research and Therapy, 33,* 49–53.

Arntz, A., Dreessen, L., & Merckelbach, H. (1991). Attention, not anxiety, influences pain. *Behavior Research and Therapy, 29,* 41–50.

Aronoff, G. M., Evans, W. O., & Enders, P. L. (1983). A review of follow-up studies of multi-disciplinary pain units. *Pain, 16,* 1–11.

Aronoff, G. M., Evans, W. O., & Enders, P. L. (1985). A review of follow-up studies in multi-disciplinary units. In G. M. Aronoff (Ed.), *Evaluation and*

269

treatment of chronic pain (pp. 511–521). Baltimore, MD: Urban and Schwarzenberg.

Aronoff, G. M., Wagner, J., & Spangler, S. (1986). Clinical interventions for pain. *Journal of Consulting and Clinical Psychology, 54,* 769–775.

Atkinson, J., & Slater, M. (1991). Prevalence, onset and risk of psychiatric disorders in men with chronic low back pain: A controlled study. *Pain, 45,* 111–121.

Bakal, D. A. (1982). *The psychobiology of chronic headache.* New York: Springer Publishing Company.

Bakal, D. A., Jen, S., & Kaganov, J. A. (1981). Cognitive-behavioral treatment of chronic headache. *Headache, 21,* 81–86.

Beals, J. (1984). Compensation recovery from injury. *Western Journal of Medicine, 40,* 233–237.

Beck, A. T., Steer, R., & Garbin, M. (1988). Psychometric properties of the Beck Depression Inventory. *Clinical Psychology Review, 8,* 77–100.

Beck, A. T., Ward, C. H., Mendelson, M., Mock, J., & Erbaugh, J. (1961). An inventory for measuring depression. *Archives of General Psychiatry, 4,* 561–571.

Beecher, H. K. (1959). *The measurement of subjective responses.* New York: Oxford University Press.

Bergner, M., Bobbitt, R. A., Carter, N. B., & Gilson, B. S. (1981). The sickness impact profile: Development and final revision of a health status measure. *Medical Care, 19,* 787–805.

Bernstein, D. A., & Borkovec, T. D. (1973). *Progressive relaxation training: A manual for helping professions.* Champaign, IL: Research Press.

Blanchard, E. B., & Ahles, T. (1990). Biofeedback therapy. In J. Bonica (Ed.), *The management of pain.* Malvern, PA: Lea & Febiger.

Blanchard, E. B., & Andrasik, F. (1982). Psychological assessment and treatment of headache: Recent developments and emerging issues. *Journal of Consulting and Clinical Psychology, 50,* 6859–6879.

Blanchard, E. B., & Andrasik, F. (1985). *The management of chronic headache: A psychological approach.* New York: Pergamon Press.

Blanchard, E. B., Andrasik, F., Ahles, T. A., Teders, S. J., & O'Keefe, D. M. (1980). Migraine and tension headache: A meta-analytic review. *Behavior Therapy, 11,* 613–631.

Blanchard, E. B., Andrasik, F., Neff, D. E., Jurish, S. E., & O'Keefe, D. M. (1981). Social validation of headache diary. *Behavior Therapist, 12,* 711–715.

Blanchard, E. B., Andrasik, F., Neff, D. E., Marina, J. G., Ahles, T. A., Jurisch, S. E., Pallmeyer, T. P., Saunders, N. L., Tedder, S. J., Baron, K. D., &

Rodichok, L. D. (1982). Biofeedback and relaxation training with three types of headache: Treatment effects and their prediction. *Journal of Consulting and Clinical Psychology, 50,* 562–575.

Block, A. (1980). Behavioral treatment of chronic pain: Variables affecting treatment efficacy. *Pain, 8,* 367–375.

Blumer, D., & Heilbronn, M. (1982). Chronic pain as a variant of depressive disease. *Journal of Nervous and Mental Disease, 170,* 381–408.

Boden, S. D., Davis, D. O., Dina, T. S., Patronas, N. J., & Wiesel, S. W. (1990). Abnormal magnetic-resonance scans of the lumbar spine in asymptomatic subjects. *The Journal of Bone and Joint Surgery, 72*-A, 403–408.

Boltz, W. (1984). The disuse syndrome. *Western Journal of Medicine, 141,* 691–694.

Bond, M. R., & Pilowsky, I. (1966). Subjective assessment of pain and its relationship to the advanced cancer. *Journal of Psychosomatic Research, 10,* 203–208.

Bonica, J. J. (1976). *Advances in neurology: International symposium on pain.* New York: Raven Press.

Bonica, J. J. (1990a). Evolution and current status of pain programs. *Journal of Pain and Symptom Management, 5,* 368–374.

Bonica, J. J. (Ed.). (1990b). *The Management of Pain.* Malvern, PA: Lea & Febiger.

Bonica, J. J., & Fordyce, W. E. (1974). Operant conditioning for chronic pain. In J. J. Bonica, P. Procacci, & C. A. Pagni (Eds.), *Recent advances in pain: Pathophysiology and clinical aspects* (pp. 299–312). Springfield, IL: C. C. Thomas.

Boston, K., Pearce, S. A., & Richardson, P. H. (1990). The Pain Cognitions Questionnaire. *Journal of Psychosomatic Research, 34,* 103–109.

Brena, S. R. (1980). Conditioned responses to treatment in chronic pain patients: Effects of compensation for work-related accidents. *Bulletin of L. A. Neurological Society, 44,* 48–52.

Brown, G. (1990). A causal analysis of chronic pain and depression. *Journal of Abnormal Psychology, 99,* 127–137.

Bryant, R. (1993). Memory for pain and affect in chronic pain patients. *Pain, 54,* 347–351.

Budzynski, T. H., Stoyva, J. M., & Adler, C. (1973). EMG Biofeedback and tension headache. *Psychosomatic Medicine, 35,* 484–496.

Cairns, D., Thomas, L., Mooney, V., & Pace, J. B. (1976). A comprehensive treatment approach to chronic low back pain. *Pain, 2,* 301–308.

Chapman, C. R. (1979). Pain: The perception of noxious events. In R. A. Sternbach (Ed.), *The psychology of pain* (pp. 169–202). New York: Raven Press.

Chapman, S. L., Brennan, S. F., & Bradford, L. A. (1981). Treatment outcome in chronic pain rehabilitation programs. *Pain, 11,* 255–268.

Cioffi, D. (1991). Beyond attentional strategies: A cognitive-perceptual model of somatic interpretation. *Psychological Bulletin, 109,* 25–41.

Derebury, J., & Tullis, W. H. (1983). Delayed recovery in patients with work compensation injuries. *Journal of Occupational Medicine, 125*(11), 829–835.

Devine, D. P., & Spanos, N. P. (1990). Effectiveness of maximally different cognitive coping strategies and expectancy in attenuation of reported pain. *Journal of Personality and Social Psychology, 58,* 672–678.

Dolce, J. J., & Crocker, M. F. (1986a). Exercise quotas, anticipatory concern, and self-efficacy expectancies in chronic pain: A preliminary report. *Pain, 24*(3), 355–365.

Dolce, J. J., & Crocker, M. F. (1986b). The prediction of outcome among chronic pain patients. *Behavior Research and Therapy, 24*(3), 313–319.

Dunnell, K., & Cartwright, A. (Eds.). (1972). *Medicine takers, prescribers and hoarders.* London: Routledge & Kegan Paul.

Dworkin, R. H., Handlin, D. S., Richlin, D. M., Brand, L., & Vannucci, C. (1985). Unravelling the effects of compensation, litigation, and employment on treatment response in chronic pain. *Pain, 23,* 49–59.

Edwards, L. C., Pearce, S. A., Turner-Stokes, L., & Jones, A. (1992). The Pain Beliefs Questionnaire: An investigation of beliefs in the causes and consequences of pain. *Pain, 51,* 267–272.

Eich, E., Rachman, S., & Lopatka, C. (1990). Affect, pain, and autobiographical memory. *Journal of Abnormal Psychology, 99,* 174–178.

Fernandez, E., & Turk, D. C. (1989). The utility of cognitive coping strategies for altering pain perception: A meta-analysis. *Pain, 38,* 123–135.

Flor, H., Behle, D., & Birbaumer, N. (1993). Assessment of pain-related cognitions in chronic pain patients. *Behavior Research and Therapy, 31,* 63–73.

Flor, H., & Birbaumer, N. (1993). Comparison of the efficacy of electromyographic biofeedback, cognitive-behavioral therapy, and conservative medical interventions in the treatment of chronic musculoskeletal pain. *Journal of Consulting and Clinical Psychology, 61,* 653–658.

Flor, H., Fydrich, T., & Turk, D. C. (1992). Efficacy of multidisciplinary pain treatment centers: A meta-analytic review. *Pain, 49,* 221–230.

Foley, K. M. (1985). Adjuvant analgesic drugs in cancer pain management. In G. M. Aronoff (Ed.), *Evaluation and treatment of chronic pain* (pp. 425–434). Baltimore, MD: Urban & Schwarzenberg.

Fordyce, W. E. (1974). Treating chronic pain by contingency management. In J. Bonica, (Ed.), *International Symposium on Pain: Advances in Neurology: Vol. 4* (pp. 538–589). New York: Raven Press.

Fordyce, W. E. (1976). *Behavioral methods for chronic pain and illness.* St. Louis: Moseby.

Fordyce, W. E., Brockway, J., Bergman, J., & Spingler, D. (1985). Acute back pain: A control group comparison of behavioral and traditional management methods. *Journal of Behavioral Medicine, 9*(2), 127–140.

Fordyce, W. E., McMahon, R., Ramweater, G., Jackins, S., Questad, K., Murphy, T., & DeLateur, B. (1981). Pain complaint: Exercise performance relationship in chronic pain. *Pain, 10,* 311–321.

Freud, S. (1893–1895). Studies on hysteria. Volume 2. In J. Strachey (Ed. and Transl.) *The standard edition of the complete psychological works of Sigmund Freud.* (1953). London: Hogarth Press.

Gamsa, A. (1990). Is emotional disturbance a precipitator or a consequence of chronic pain? *Pain, 42,* 183–195.

Gil, K. M., Williams, D., Keefe, F. J., & Beckham, J. C. (1990). The relationship of negative thoughts to pain and psychological distress. *Behavior Therapy, 21,* 349–362.

Gottlieb, H., Streit, L. C., Koller, R., Maderasky, Z., Hockersmith, V., Kellman, M., & Wagner, J. (1977). Comprehensive rehabilitation of patients having chronic low back pain. *Archives of Physical Medicine Rehabilitation, 58,* 101–108.

Guck, T. P., Skultety, F. M., Meilman, P. W., & Dowed, E. T. (1985). Multidisciplinary pain center follow-up study: Evaluation with a no-treatment control group. *Pain, 21*(3), 295–307.

Hamburgen, M. E., & Jennings, C. A. (1985). Failure of predictive scale in identifying patients who may benefit from pain management programs: Follow-up data. *Pain, 23,* 253–258.

Hathaway, D. (1986). Effects of preoperative instruction on postoperative outcomes: A meta-analysis. *Nursing Research, 35,* 269–275.

Hawton, K., Salkovskis, P., Kirk, J., & Clark, D. (Eds.). (1989). *Cognitive behavior therapy for psychiatric problems.* Oxford: Oxford University Press.

Haythornthwaite, J., Sieber, W., & Kerns, R. (1991). Depression and the chronic pain experience. *Pain, 46,* 177–184.

Holroyd, K. A., & Penzien, D. B. (1990). Pharmacological versus non-pharmacological prophylaxis of recurrent migraine headache: A meta-analytic review of clinical trials. *Pain, 42,* 1–13.

Holroyd, K. A. (1985). Recurrent migraine and tension headache. In K. Holroyd & T. Creer (Eds.), *Self-management of physical disease: Developments in health, psychology, and behavioral medicine* (pp. 373–405). New York: Academic Press.

Holroyd, K. A., Andrasik, F., & Wesbrook, T. (1977). Cognitive control of tension headache. *Cognitive Therapy/Research, 1,* 121–133.

Holzman, A., & Turk, D. (Eds.). (1986). *Pain management: A handbook of psychological treatment approaches.* New York: Pergamon Press.

Hunter, M. (1983). The headache scale: A new approach to the assessment of headache pain based on pain descriptors. *Pain, 16,* 361–373.

Hunter, M., Philips, H. C., & Rachman, S. (1979). Memory for pain. *Pain, 6,* 35–46.

Jacob, M. C., Kerns, R. D., Rosenberg, R., & Haythornthwaite, J. (1993). Chronic pain: Intrusion and accommodation. *Behavior Research and Therapy, 31,* 519–527.

Jacobson, E. (1938). *Progressive relaxation.* Chicago: Chicago University Press.

Jahanshahi, M., Hunter, M., & Philips, C. (1986). The headache scale: An examination of its reliability and validity. *Headache, 26*(2), 76–82.

Jensen, M., Brant-Zawadzki, M., Obuchowski, N., Modic, M., Malkasian, D., & Ross, J. (1994). Magnetic resonance imaging of the lumbar spine in people without back pain. *New England Journal of Medicine, 331,* 69–73.

Jensen, M. P., Karoly, P., & Braver, S. (1986). The measurement of clinical pain intensity: A comparison of six methods. *Pain, 27,* 117–126.

Jensen, M. P., Turner, J. A., & Romano, J. M. (1994). Correlates of improvement in multi-disciplinary treatment of chronic pain. *Journal of Consulting and Clinical Psychology, 62,* 172–179.

Johnson, F. H. (1973). The effects of accurate expectations on the sensory and distress components of pain. *Journal of Personality and Social Psychology, 27,* 261–275.

Johnson, F. H., & Leventhal, H. (1974). Effects of accurate expectations and behavioral instructions on reactions during a noxious medical examination. *Journal of Personality and Social Psychology, 29,* 710–718.

Keefe, F., Crisson, J., Urban, R., & Williams, J. (1990). Analyzing chronic low back pain: The relative contribution of pain coping strategies. *Pain, 40,* 293–301.

Krusen, E. M., & Ford, D. E. (1958). Compensation factors in low back injury. *Journal of American Medical Association, 166,* 1128–1133.

Lander, J., & Hodgins, M. (1992). Children's pain predictions and memories. *Behavior Research and Therapy, 30,* 117–124.

Lang, P. J. (1978) Fear reduction and fear behavior: Problems in treating the construct. In J. M. Shlien (Ed.), *Research in psychotherapy* (pp. 90–102). Washington, DC: American Psychological Association.

Latimer, P. (1982). External contingency management of chronic pain: A critical review of the evidence. *American Journal of Psychiatry, 139,* 1308–1312.

Lefebvre, M. F. (1981). Cognitive distortion and cognitive errors in depressed psychiatric and low back pain patients. *Journal of Consulting and Clinical Psychology, 49,* 517–525.

Leventhal, H. (1992). I know distraction works even though it doesn't! *Health Psychology, 11,* 208–209.

Lichstein, K. (1988). *Clinical Relaxation Strategies.* New York: Wiley.

Linton, S. J. (1985). Relationship between activity and chronic back pain. *Pain, 21,* 289–294.

Linton, S. J., Hellsing, A., & Andersson, S. (1993). A controlled study of the effects of an early intervention on acute musculoskeletal pain problems. *Pain, 54,* 353–359.

Linton, S. J. (1986). Behavioral remediation of chronic pain: A status report. *Pain, 24*(2), 125–143.

Magni, G., & Caldieron, C. (1990). Chronic musculoskeletal pain and depressive symptoms in the general population: An analysis of the 1st National Health and Nutrition Examination Survey. *Pain, 43,* 299–307.

McCaul, K. D., & Mallot, J. M. (1984). Distraction and coping with pain. *Psychological Bulletin, 95*(3), 516–533.

Meichenbaum, D., & Turk, D. (1990). *Facilitating treatment adherence.* New York: Plenum Press.

Melzack, R. (1975). The McGill Pain Questionnaire: Major properties and scoring methods. *Pain, 1,* 277–299.

Melzack, R. (Ed.). (1983). *Pain measurement and assessment.* New York: Raven Press.

Melzack, R. (1989). Phantom limbs, the self and the brain. *Canadian Psychology, 30,* 1–16.

Melzack, R. (1993). Pain: Past, present and future. *Canadian Journal of Experimental Psychology, 47,* 615–629.

Melzack, R., & Loeser, J. D. (1978). Phantom body pain in paraplegics: Evidence for a central "pattern generating mechanism" for pain. *Pain, 4,* 195–210.

Melzack, R., & Perry, C. (1975). Self-regulation of pain in the use of alpha-feedback and hypnotic training for the control of chronic pain. *Experimental Neurology, 46,* 252–269.

Melzack, R., & Torgerson, W. S. (1971). The language of pain. *Anaesthesiology, 34,* 50–59.

Melzack, R., & Wall, P. (1965). Pain mechanisms: A new theory. *Science, 150,* 971–979.

Melzack, R., & Wall, P. (1982). Acute pain in an emergency clinic. *Pain, 14,* 33–43.

Melzack, R., & Wall, P. (1988). *The challenge of pain.* Harmondsworth, Middlesex, England: Penguin Books.

Melzack, R., Wall, P., & Ty, T. C. (1982). Acute pain in an emergency clinic. *Pain, 14,* 263–269.

Merskey, H. (Ed.). (1980). *Psychiatric illness: Diagnosis, management and treatment for general practitioners and students.* London: Bailliere Tindal.

Morley, S. (1993). Vivid memory for "everyday" pains. *Pain, 55,* 55–62.

Moskowitz, M. A., & Cutrer, F. M. (1993). Sumatriptan: A receptor targeted treatment for migraine. *Annual Review of Medicine, 44,* 145–154.

Moss, R. A. (1986). The role of learning history in current sick-role behavior and assertion. *Behavior Research and Therapy, 24*(6), 681–685.

Newman, R. I., Seres, J. L., & Yossep, L. P. (1983). Multi-disciplinary treatment of chronic pain: Long-term follow-up of low back pain patients. *Pain, 4,* 283–292.

Oral Sumatriptan International Multiple-Dose Study Group. (1991). Evaluation of a multiple-dose regimen of oral sumatriptan for the acute treatment of migraine. Eighth Migraine Trust International Symposium: Sumatriptan: From molecule to man. In *European Neurology, 31,* 316–333.

Pearce, J., & Morley, S. (1989). An experimental investigation of the construct validity of the McGill Pain Questionnaire. *Pain, 39,* 115–121.

Pearce, S. (1983). A review of cognitive-behavioral methods for the treatment of chronic pain. *Journal of Psychosomatic Research, 27*(5), 431–440.

Philips, H. C. (1983). The nature and treatment of tension headache. In K. D. Craig & R. J. McMahon (Eds.), *Advances in clinical behavior therapy* (pp. 211–232). New York: Brunner/Mazel.

Philips, H. C. (1987a). The effects of behavioral treatment on chronic pain. *Behavior Research and Therapy, 25,* 365–378.

Philips, H. C. (1987b). Thoughts provoked by pain. *Behavior Research and Therapy, 27,* 469–474.

Philips, H. C. (1987c). Avoidance behavior and its role in sustaining chronic pain. *Behavior Research and Therapy, 25,* 273–280.

Philips, H. C. (1988). Changing chronic pain experience. *Pain, 32,* 165–172.

Philips, H. C., & Grant, L. (1991a). The evolution of chronic back pain problems. *Behavior Research and Therapy, 29,* 435–441.

Philips, H. C., & Grant, L. (1991b). Acute back pain: A psychological analysis. *Behavior Research and Therapy, 29,* 429–434.

Philips, H. C., & Hunter, M. (1981). Pain behavior in headache sufferers. *Behavior Analysis and Modification, 4,* 257–265.

Philips, H. C., & Jahanshahi, M. (1985). The effects of persistent pain: The chronic headache sufferer. *Pain, 21,* 163–176.

Philips, H. C., & Jahanshahi, M. (1986). The components of pain behavior report. *Behavior Research and Therapy, 24*(2), 117–125.

Pilowsky, I., & Katsikitis, M. (1994). A classification of illness behavior in pain clinic patients. *Pain, 57,* 91–94.

Rachman, S. (1990). *Fear and courage* (2nd ed.). New York: W. H. Freeman.

Rachman, S. (1993). A critique of cognitive therapy for anxiety disorders. *Journal of Behavior Therapy and Experimental Psychiatry, 24,* 279–288.

Rachman, S., & Arntz, A. (1991). The overprediction and underprediction of pain. *Clinical Psychology Review, 11,* 339–355.

Rachman, S., & Bichard, S. (1988). The overprediction of fear. *Clinical Psychology Review, 8,* 303–312.

Rachman, S., & Eyrl, K. (1989). Predicting and remembering recurrent pain. *Behavior Research and Therapy, 27,* 621–635.

Rachman, S., & Hodgson, R. (1974). Synchrony and desynchrony in fear and avoidance. *Behavior Research and Therapy, 12,* 311–318.

Rachman, S., & Philips, H. C. (1980). *Psychology and Behavioral Medicine.* New York: Cambridge University Press.

Rachman, S., & Wilson, G. (1980). *The effects of psychological therapy.* Oxford: Pergamon Press.

Roberts, A. H., & Reinhardt, L. (1980). The behavioral management of chronic pain: Long-term follow-up with comparison groups. *Pain, 8,* 151–162.

Romano, J. M., & Turner, J. A. (1985). Chronic pain and depression: Does the evidence support a relationship? *Psychological Bulletin, 97,* 18–34.

Rose, F. C. (1993). Sumatriptan: An overview. *Headache Quarterly, 4,* 37–41.

Salovey, P., Smith, A. F., Turk, D. C., Jobe, J. B., & Willis, G. B. (in press). The accuracy of memory for pain: Not so bad most of the time.

Sarkis, E., & Turner, J. A. (1982). Self-report versus actual use of medication in chronic pain patients. *Pain, 12,* 285–294.

Seres, J. L., Paynter, J. R., & Newman, R. I. (1981). Multi-disciplinary treatment of chronic pain at the Northwest Pain Centre. In L. Lorenz & K. Ng (Eds.), *New approach to chronic pain: A review of multi-disciplinary pain clinics and pain centers* (NIDA Research Monograph No. 36). Washington, DC: U.S. Government Printing Office.

Sheftell, F. D., & Weeks, R. E. (1994). Subcutaneous sumatriptan in a clinical setting: The first 100 consecutive patients with acute migraine in a tertiary care center. *Headache, 34,* 67–72.

Smith, W. B., & Safer, M. A. (1993). Effects of present pain level on recall of chronic pain and medication use. *Pain, 55,* 355–361.

Spielberger, C. S. (1983). *Manual for the state-trait anxiety inventory.* Palo Alto, CA: Consulting Psychologists Press, Inc.

Spinhoven, P., & Linssen, A. (1991). Behavioral treatment of chronic low back pain, I: Relation of coping strategy use to outcome. *Pain, 45,* 29–34.

Stenn, P. G., Mothersill, K. J., & Brooke, R. I. (1979). Biofeedback and cognitive behavioral approach to the treatment of myofacial pain dysfunction syndrome. *Behavior Therapy, 10,* 29–36.

Sternbach, R. A. (1974). *Pain patients: traits and treatment.* New York: Academic Press.

Suis, J., & Fletcher, B. (1985). The relative efficacy of avoidant and non-avoidant coping strategies: Meta analysis. *Health Psychology, 4*(3), 249–289.

Sullivan, M., & D'Eon, J. (1990). Relation between catastrophizing and depression in chronic pain patients. *Journal of American Psychology, 99,* 260–263.

Sullivan, M. J. L., Reesor, K., Mikail, S., & Fisher, R. (1992). The treatment of depression in chronic low back pain: Review and recommendations. *Pain, 50,* 5–13.

Suls, J., & Wan, C. K. (1989). Effects of sensory and procedural information on coping with stressful medical procedures and pain. A meta-analysis. *Journal of Consulting and Clinical Psychology, 57,* 372–379.

Tan, S. Y. (1982). Cognitive and cognitive behavioral methods for pain control: A selective review. *Pain, 12,* 201–228.

Tansey, M. J., & Pilgrim, A. J. (1993). Long-term experience with sumatriptan in the treatment of migraine. *European Neurology, 33,* 310–315.

Teasdale, J. D., & Barnard, P. J. (1993). *Affect, cognition and change: Remodelling depressive thought.* Hillsdale, NJ: Lawrence Erlbaum.

Tomlin, P., Thyer, B., Curtis, G., Nesse, R., Camero, D., & Wright, P. (1984). Standardization of the FSS. *Journal of Behavior Therapy and Experimental Psychiatry, 15,* 123–126.

Trief, P., & Stein, N. (1985). Pending litigation and rehabilitation outcome of chronic back pain. *Archives of Physical Medicine and Rehabilitation, 66*(2), 95–99.

Turk, D. C., & Flor, H. (1984). Ideological theories in treatment for chronic back pain II: Psychological models and interventions. *Pain, 19,* 209–233.

Turk, D. C., Meichenbaum, D., & Genest, M. (1983). *Pain and behavioral medicine: A cognitive behavioral perspective.* New York: Guilford Publications.

Turk, D. C., & Rudy, T. E. (1992). Cognitive factors and persistent pain: A glimpse into Pandora's box. *Cognitive Therapy and Research, 16,* 99–122.

Turk, D. C., & Rudy, T. E. (1987). Towards a comprehensive assessment of chronic pain patients: A multiaxial approach. *Behavior Research and Therapy, 25,* 237–249.

Turk, D. C., Wack, J. T., & Kearns, R. D. (1985). An empirical examination of the "pain behavior" construct. *Journal of Behavioral Medicine, 8,* 119–130.

Turner, J. A. (1983). A comparison of group progressive relaxation training and cognitive behavioral group therapy for chronic low back pain. *Journal of Consulting and Clinical Psychology, 67,* 657–765.

Turner, J. A., & Chapman, C. R. (1982). Psychological interventions for chronic pain: A critical review, I and II. *Pain, 12,* 1–46.

Turner, J. A., Deyo, R. A., Loeser, J. D., Von Korff, M., & Fordyce, W. E. (1994). The importance of placebo effects in pain treatment and research. *Journal of the American Medical Association, 271,* 1609–1614.

Turner, J. A., & Jensen, M. P. (1993). Efficacy of cognitive therapy for chronic low back pain. *Pain, 52,* 169–177.

Turner, J., & Romano, J. (1990). Cognitive behavioral therapy. In J. Bonica (Ed.), *The management of pain.* Malvern, PA: Lea & Febiger.

Turner, J. A., Colgyn, D. A. (1982). Drug utilization patterns in chronic pain patients. *Pain, 12,* 357–363.

Vlaeyen, J., & Pernots, D. (1990). Assessment of the components of observed chronic pain behavior: The Checklist for Interpersonal Pain Behavior (CHIP). *Pain, 43,* 337–347.

Waddell, G., & Newton, M. (1993). A Fear-Avoidance Beliefs Questionnaire (FABQ) and the role of fear-avoidance beliefs in chronic low back pain and disability. *Pain, 52,* 157–168.

Wall, P. D., & Melzack, R. (1989). *Textbook of pain.* New York: Churchill Livingstone.

Wall, P. W. (1979). On the relation of injury to pain. *Pain, 6,* 253–264.

Walmsley, P. N. H., & Brockopp, G. W. (1992). The role of prior pain experience and expectations on post-operative pain. *Journal of Pain and Symptom Management, 7,* 34–37.

Weisenberg, M. (1980). Understanding pain phenomena. In S. Rachman (Ed.), *Contributions to medical psychology, Vol. 2* (pp. 79–111). Elmsford, New York: Pergamon Press.

Weisenberg, M. (1987). Psychological intervention for the control of pain. *Behavior Research and Therapy, 25,* 301–312.

Weisenberg, M., Aviram, O., Wolf, Y., & Raphael, I. N. (1984). Relevant and irrelevant anxiety in the reaction to pain. *Pain, 20*(4), 371–385.

White, B., & Saunders, S. H. (1985). Differential effects on pain and mood in chronic pain with time versus pain contingent medication delivery. *Behavior Therapy, 60*(1), 28–39.

Wiesel, S. W., Tsourmas, N., Feffer, H. L., Citrin, C. M., & Patronas, N. (1984). A study of computer-assisted tomography. I. The incidence of positive CAT scans in an asymptomatic group of patients. *Spine, 9,* 549–551.

Williams, D. A., & Thorn, B. E. (1989). An empirical assessment of pain beliefs. *Pain, 36,* 351–358.

Williams, J., & Spitzer, R. (1982). Research diagnostic criteria and DSM-III: An annotated comparison. *Archives of General Psychiatry, 39,* 1283–1289.

Wilson, G. T. (1984). Fear reduction methods. In G. T. Wilson, C. Franks, K. Bownell, & P. Kendall (Eds.), *Annual review of psychology, Vol. 9* (pp. 95–131). New York: Guilford Press.

Wittig, R. M. (1982). Disturbed sleep in chronic pain. *Journal of Nervous and Mental Disorders, 170,* 429–431.

Wolpe, J. (1958). *Psychotherapy by reciprocal inhibition.* Stanford, CA: Stanford University Press.

Wuitchik, M., Bakal, D., & Lipshitz, J. (1990). Relationships between pain, cognitive activity and epidural analgesia during labor. *Pain, 41,* 125–132.

Zarkowska, E., & Philips, H. C. (1985). A pain behavior questionnaire. Unpublished manuscript.

Index

SP Springer Publishing Company

PSYCHOLOGICAL VULNERABILITY TO CHRONIC PAIN
Roy C. Grzesiak, PhD & Donald S. Ciccone, PhD

In this volume, prominent scientist-practitioners examine the psychological and psychosocial factors that influence risk and vulnerability to disabling and persistent pain and suggest ways in which these factors can be reduced.

The expert editors and contributors consider the impact of a wide range of nonorganic variables on pain, in order to encourage further exploration of this important topic. Featured in the Appendix is a reprint of a classic article on psychogenic pain by George L. Engel.

> *Psychological Vulnerability to Chronic Pain*
>
> Roy C. Grzesiak, PhD
> Donald S. Ciccone, PhD
>
> *Springer Publishing Company*
> SP

Contents:

- The Matrix of Vulnerability, *R.C. Grzesiak*
- Somatizing as a Risk Factor for Chronic Pain, *S.F. Dworkin, L. Wilson, and D.L. Massoth*
- Muscle Overuse and Posture as Factors in the Development and Maintenance of Chronic Musculoskeletal Pain, *S.J. Middaugh, W.G. Kee, and J. Nicholson*
- Pain Proneness in Children: Toward a New Conceptual Model, *J.E. Goodman, Y. Gidron, and P.J. McGrath*
- Chronic Daily Headache and the Elusive Nature of Somatic Awareness, *D. Bakal, S. Demjen, and P.N. Duckro*
- Attachment and Pain, *D.J. Anderson and R.H. Hines*
- Psychological Vulnerability to Chronic Dysfunctional Pain: A Critical Review, *D.S. Ciccone and V. Lenzi* • "Psychogenic" Pain and the Pain-prone Patient, *G.L. Engel*

1994   248pp   0-8261-8070-1   hardcover

536 Broadway, New York, NY 10012-3955 • (212) 431-4370 • Fax (212) 941-7842

$ *Springer Publishing Company*

RELATIONSHIP-CENTERED COUNSELING
An Integation of Art and Science

Eugene W. Kelly, Jr., PhD

In this insightful and well-written volume, the author courageously defines counseling as both art and science. He explains that effective counseling is based on the core counselor-client relationship and requires a unique integration of humanism and technical knowledge. From this conceptual perspective, the author expertly offers practical guidelines to aid counselors in their craft. This book will appeal to counselors, psychologists, psychotherapists, social workers, psychiatrists, family therapists and academics involved in counselor training.

Contents:

- Counseling as Passionate Virtuosity
- The Humanity of the Counselor
- Modeling the Client: Core Principles of Humanness
- Modeling the Client: Culture, Development, Interaction, Reality
- The Counseling Relationship: Integrative Center, and In-Depth Field of The Counseling Art
- The Counseling Relationship: Introductory Concepts and The Paratherapeutic Component
- The Counseling Relationship: The Direct Therapeutic Relational Component
- Relationship Extended: Scientific and Technical Expertise in Counseling
- The Counseling Art: A Look to the Future

1994 324pp 0-8261-8210-0 hardcover

536 Broadway, New York, NY 10012-3955 • (212) 431-4370 • Fax (212) 941-7842

$\boxed{\text{S}}$ *Springer Publishing Company*

LOGOTHERAPY FOR THE HELPING PROFESSIONAL
Meaningful Social Work

David Guttmann, DSW

In this useful resource, the author explains the pioneering work of Dr. Viktor Frankl and his theories of logotherapy. This volume will enable helping professionals to supplement traditional methods of psychotherapy with logotherapy techniques in order to improve their effectiveness through clearer understanding of their clients' problems. Professionals can then derive greater personal meaning and satisfaction from their work, thereby lessening the potential for stress and burnout. This volume addresses therapists, clinical social workers, and counselors.

Contents:

I: Major Concepts in Logotherapy. The Development of Logotherapy • Logotherapy and Psychoanalysis: Similarities and Differences • The Noetic or Spiritual Dimension • The "Tragic Triad": Logotherapy's Attitude to Guilt, Suffering, and Death

II: Logotherapeutic Treatment and Application. Paradoxical Intention as a Special Logotherapeutic Technique • "Dereflection" as Counteracting Behavior • Other Logotherapeutic Techniques • The "Socratic Dialogue" Logotherapy's Main Tool in Helping Seekers Search for Meaning

III. Research in the Service of Logotherapy. Research on Major Logotherapeutic Concepts • Further Developments in Logotherapeutic Research

1995 320pp 0-8261-9020-0 hardcover

536 Broadway, New York, NY 10012-3955 • (212) 431-4370 • Fax (212) 941-7842

Ⓢ *Springer Publishing Company*

BREAST CANCER
A Psychological Treatment Manual

Sandra Haber, PhD, Editor

This volume, originally published by the Division of Independent Practice of the American Psychological Association, was designed to educate and involve therapists and counselors in the psychological treatment of patients and their families. This manual represents a collaborative venture of 10 women psychologists who address the emotional responses of breast cancer patients, families, and caretakers, as well as the psychological, social, and behavioral factors that may influence cancer morbidity and mortality.

Contents:

I: Medical Aspects of Breast Cancer. Medical Treatment of Breast Cancer • The Relationships Among Patient, Physician and Psychologist

II: Stages of Breast Cancer: Patient's Experience and Treatment. Psychological Reactions to Diagnosis and Treatment • Psychological Reactions to Posttreatment • Recurrence and Terminal Illness

III: Psychotherapy with the Breast Cancer Patient. The Patient-Psychologist Relationship • Support Groups/Group Therapy • Special Populations: High Risk Women, Lesbian Women, Women of Poverty and Ethnicity, and Older Women • Countertransference

IV: Psychological Interventions with the Family. Husbands and Significant Others • Helping the Children

V: Interventions and Resources. Specific Interventions • Research on the Effectiveness of Psychological Interventions • Resources • Selected Medical Glossary

1994   160pp   0-8261-8790-0   hardcover

536 Broadway, New York, NY 10012-3955 • (212) 431-4370 • Fax (212) 941-7842